Mind

—— over ——

Malignancy

LIVING WITH CANCER

Wayne D. Gersh, Ph.D.

William L. Golden, Ph.D.

& David M. Robbins, Ph.D.

New Harbinger Publications

Publisher's Note

This publication is designed to provide accurate and authoritative information in regard to the subject matter covered. It is sold with the understanding that the publisher is not engaged in rendering psychological, financial, legal, or other professional services. If expert assistance or counseling is needed, the services of a competent professional should be sought.

Distributed in the U.S.A. by Publishers Group West; in Canada by Raincoast Books; in Great Britain by Airlift Book Company, Ltd.; in South Africa by Real Books, Ltd.; in Australia by Boobook; and in New Zealand by Tandem Press.

Copyright © 1997 by Wayne D. Gersh, Ph.D.; William L. Golden, Ph.D.;
and David M. Robbins, Ph.D.
New Harbinger Publications, Inc.
5674 Shattuck Avenue
Oakland, CA 94609

Cover design by Lightbourne Images © 1997.
Text design by Tracy Marie Powell.
Edited by Carole Honeychurch.

Library of Congress Catalog Card Number: 97-66076

ISBN 1-57224-082-2

Printed in the United States of America on recycled paper.

New Harbinger Publications' Web site address: www.newharbinger.com.

10   9   8   7   6   5   4   3   2   1

We wish to dedicate this book to our patients, who inspired, taught, and encouraged us throughout this endeavor.

We would also like to thank our wives, Barbara Gersh, Carolyn McCarthy-Golden, and Helene Robbins, for their support and patience during the writing of this book.

Contents

Foreword

We have been counseling and helping cancer patients cope with their illness for the last seventeen years. Our clinical work has been described in detail in *Psychological Treatment of Cancer Patients: A Cognitive-Behavioral Approach,* a treatment manual that has been widely used by hospitals, treatment centers, and practitioners in private practice.

The inspiration for this book came as the result of the very favorable response to our first book. Many of our colleagues and patients urged us to write a book that could be used by you, the cancer survivor; and because this book is for the layperson, we chose to write it in a conversational style, without all the references that can be found in our textbook.

Additionally, many of our patients have told us that most of the other books written to help cancer patients are long on inspiration but short on technique. We believe that our book is unique in that it combines inspiration with specific psychological skills. These skills have been shown to be quite effective in helping cancer patients learn how to take control of their lives and their illness. This is one of the first books to specifically address questions raised by most cancer patients, questions like, "How can I manage my feelings?" and "What can I do to cope with this illness?"

If you are interested in researching the clinical and experimental evidence that has influenced our writing, you can refer to our textbook. We hope that we have presented the essence of that material here in a way that is easy for you to read and practical for you to use.

We want to thank all of our patients—the people who taught us most of what we needed to know in order to write this book. We've done everything possible to protect their anonymity: Their names have been changed and we altered details of their lives, which, if included, might disclose their identities. The one exception is not a patient, but our co-author, Dr. David Robbins. David was diagnosed with brain cancer in 1995 and used the techniques in this book not only to survive, but to improve the quality of his life and attain goals such as the completion of this book. We hope that all of these stories will be an inspiration for you and will encourage you to move forward, using the tools we offer, so that you too can experience mind over malignancy.

Wayne D. Gersh, Ph.D.
White Plains, NY

William L. Golden, Ph.D.
New York, NY

David M. Robbins, Ph.D.
West Nyack, NY

Empowerment: How This Book Can Help You Gain Control

In this chapter, we will give you a preview of the techniques that you as a cancer survivor can use for taking more control of your emotions, your behavior, and your life. These techniques can be used to control anxiety, depression, and pain. They can help you set goals, solve problems, overcome grief, and resume a normal life.

As we mentioned in the foreword, one of the authors, Dr. David Robbins, was diagnosed with brain cancer in 1995. As difficult as this has been for us, it has given us a special outlook on writing a book about cancer. We felt that we had the opportunity to write from a very personal perspective and were not only able to tell you what worked with our patients, but also what worked for one of us.

Revising Your Priorities

Dr. Robbins knew that he was going to fight the illness with the techniques in this book, but what he learned using these tools was how important his enjoyment of life and its simple pleasures were to him. His response to this realization was to eliminate those people and issues that he now knew where not helpful or important to him. Prior to his illness, David often felt that he had to work very long hours in order to be successful. He decided to change his priorities from working long hours to spending more time with his family. He also decided he did not have to get upset about or spend time with people who unduly frustrated him. You may realize that now that you have cancer, you may not want to do the same things that you did prior to the illness. That's okay!

> *Sometimes it takes a traumatic event like a serious illness or accident for us to examine and evaluate our priorities.*

So many of us waste our lives doing things we don't want to do and being with people we don't like. Sometimes it takes a traumatic event like a serious illness or accident for us to examine and evaluate our priorities. We sometimes assume that we have to act a certain way regardless of how we feel. Sometimes we do have to conform to society's demands, like working for a living. But we don't have to live to work! We have more options than we realize. It makes sense for all of us to ask ourselves the following question: "If I had only one more year to live, how would I want to live it?" We are not advocating that you should be irresponsible or selfish, and quit your job or leave your family in order to make the most of your life. We recommend that you question assumptions that may lead to unhappiness. These may include: "I have to work just as hard even though I have cancer"; "I can't change my job because I have cancer"; "I can't have fun because I have cancer"; "I can't go on vacation because I have cancer"; "I can't spend money because I have cancer"; "I shouldn't express my feelings to family and friends even if they disappoint me because now I'm a burden to them."

David chose to work less as a result of evaluating what was important to him. Some people don't have that choice. Illnesses, such as cancer, can impose real limitations. It's not helpful or realistic to deny those limitations or try to wish them away. Sometimes it's necessary and helpful to accept limitations—you can still enjoy life, but you may have to do it in a different way. That can involve enjoying simple pleasures such as listening to music, reading your favorite author, or spending time with your family. Dwelling on your illness can prevent you from enjoying simple pleasures like these. It's only natural that you will feel grief, sadness, and anxiety about your illness. We cannot eliminate those emotions for you, but we will teach you how to cope with them. This will enable you to make the most of your situation.

Your Ability to Change

Making lifestyle changes can help you to feel more in control of your life. People are also more capable of fighting cancer when they learn to be more assertive, independent, and to clarify what is meaningful in life. Focusing on your strengths encourages a positive outlook and provides you with a sense of empowerment. Cancer patients are often led to believe that they are incapable of leading a normal life. You *can* make changes in your life. You can learn to be more assertive and express your feelings. You can set new goals and continue to work on your old ones. Believe in yourself. Hope is engendered by setting and pursuing goals. Some patients are reluctant to set goals for the future out of fear that they will not be around to accomplish them. But the quality of your life will be improved if you pursue goals, regardless of how long you live. In fact, some people assert that you are more likely to live longer if you are active and continue to pursue goals. Later in the book we will teach you how to establish meaningful goals.

Setting goals and maintaining a positive outlook are important factors in coping with some of the troubling emotional issues that a cancer diagnosis can bring up. Anxiety is a natural reaction to a life-threatening situation and is a problem we've helped many patients cope with by using the techniques in this book.

Lucy: Coping with Anxiety

Lucy is a typical example of "mind over malignancy." Her case illustrates how you can use your mind to change your feelings,

> *Setting goals and maintaining a positive outlook are important factors in coping with some of the troubling emotional issues that a cancer diagnosis can bring up.*

your actions, your physical well-being, and the quality of your life. Using the methods in this book, she attained many benefits. She overcame her depression and anxiety, was able to continue her chemotherapy by controlling nausea and vomiting, and resumed a normal lifestyle. She was referred by her oncologist after her surgery for breast cancer. Her oncologist made the referral to one of the authors, Dr. Wayne Gersh, who was aware of the benefits of cognitive-behavior therapy in the treatment of depression and for control of the side effects of chemotherapy such as nausea and vomiting.

When Lucy first came to therapy she was terrified of her chemotherapy side effects. She realized that she needed chemotherapy, but unfortunately she was not responsive to antinausea medication, and was therefore in great danger of discontinuing her treatment. When Lucy's oncologist first recommended a psychologist she was very insulted and asked, "Do you think I'm crazy?" The oncologist explained that cognitive-behavior therapy was very effective for managing the side effects of chemotherapy, which are very real and not necessarily psychological. He also explained that depression as a result of a life-threatening illness is very natural.

Lucy was depressed because she felt hopeless about getting the treatment that she needed. She also felt terribly ashamed and cowardly for not wanting to go through the chemotherapy. The treatments had begun to cause a deterioration in her quality of life. Each chemotherapy session involved her being hospitalized for at least a week because the side effects were so debilitating. This interfered with her work schedule and her social life, plunging her even further into depression.

The first thing that Dr. Gersh did was to assure Lucy that these reactions were very common and understandable given her situation. He pointed out to Lucy that her belief that she was hopeless and cowardly were attitudes that made her depressed and anxious. He taught her that she could reduce some of her depression by realizing she was not a coward and that it was understandable that she would be scared given her circumstances. Furthermore, he reassured her that she was not hopeless—her symptoms were treatable. And to help her with her physical symptoms as well as her emotional ones, Wayne taught Lucy relaxation techniques.

Relaxation and imagery techniques reduce anxiety and stress and are very effective in controlling chemotherapy side effects, such as nausea and vomiting, even when antinausea medications are ineffective. These techniques produce a calming effect that reduces the possibility of an upset stomach. Some relaxation techniques such as pleasant imagery can help block out negative anxiety-producing thoughts such as: "The chemotherapy is going to make me sick—I can't stand it"; "I'll never be able to go through this"; or "I'm such a coward."

Lucy was responsive to the relaxation and imagery techniques and was therefore able to complete her chemotherapy treatments. She reported that she had a marked reduction in feelings of nausea and anxiety. Even before these improvements, she became less self-critical and more hopeful in general. She was able to resume a normal work schedule and social life.

Lucy is an example of a patient who learned how to take control of her life despite having cancer. She faced her fears and learned to control symptoms that would have prevented her from getting the treatment she needed. She went from feeling helpless and hopeless to feeling empowered. Throughout the book we will describe how you can use techniques for controlling anxiety and depression, and in chapter 4, we will show you how you can learn to control chemotherapy side effects.

Bertha: Dealing with Severe Depression

Frequently, a patient's anxiety level is compounded by severe depression. Extreme hopelessness, feelings of self-pity, and a conviction that you are powerless to fight can instill depression with a tragic result—you simply give up. Through the techniques in this book many people have regained their hopeful outlook and shed the depression that corrupted their enjoyment of life and threatened their physical well-being.

Bertha, upon hearing that she had a cancerous tumor that has a high cure rate, immediately thought, "Things are hopeless. I might as well give up and die." Her oncologist referred her to Dr. Bill Golden because she became severely depressed. Bill explained to Bertha that the reason that she became so depressed was not simply because of her diagnosis. Having cancer is cause for stress, concern, and grief. But getting severely depressed was only going to make things worse and could be avoided.

Bill agreed that there was nothing positive about having cancer. Nevertheless, Bertha could still use positive and rational thinking to cope with her illness. At first, Bertha was resistant to looking at her illness in a different manner. Bill was understanding about how hard it is to think differently about cancer, but offered many examples of how other patients were successful in reducing their depression by using cognitive therapy. He suggested that she had nothing to lose by trying this approach.

"Bertha, it's only natural that you would be upset about having cancer. Most cancer patients go through a great deal of anxiety and depression as a result of their illness. But, perhaps I can help you to feel less depressed. Many of my patients initially respond to their diagnoses by feeling hopeless and powerless. With help they were able to turn this around. You really have nothing to lose by trying out these techniques. Let's see if they can help you, like they helped so many other people."

Bertha agreed she had nothing to lose but was unsure about how Bill would go about helping her. "If I feel hopeless, won't I be too discouraged to use any of the techniques you have to offer me?"

Bill explained how hopelessness is a function of negative thinking. "The reason you feel hopeless is because you are assuming you won't respond to your medical treatment. As you've told me, when you first learned you had cancer, your automatic thoughts were: 'It's hopeless, I might as well give up and die.' Those thoughts are the reason you feel hopeless. You're still thinking that way, despite what your oncologist told you about your prognosis. Could you tell me again what he said?"

"He said that I have a very good chance of surviving. My type of cancer has a high cure rate."

"Do you remind yourself of that?" asked Bill.

"I guess not," Bertha acknowledged.

"This is where cognitive therapy can help. Cognitive therapy has been found to be the most effective treatment for depression, other than antidepressant medication. We have already accomplished the first steps of cognitive therapy. We identified the negative thoughts that are causing you to feel depressed, and we have some coping thoughts that you could use to fight your feelings of hopelessness. Whenever you feel hopeless, you could remind yourself of what the oncologist told you about your chances. We call those reminders *coping self-statements*. Coping self-statements are rational thoughts that you use whenever your negative thoughts are getting the best of you. So, Bertha, what could you tell yourself whenever you are feeling depressed?"

Together, Bertha and Bill came up with the following coping thoughts: "My doctor has assured me that my cancer is highly treatable. I'm going to go through the chemotherapy and I will survive." By repeating these coping statements to herself when she felt negative Bertha gradually became more hopeful and less depressed.

Many patients like Lucy and Bertha learn to cope with their illness and return to normal functioning. This is not always the case. Some cancer patients have had to learn to live life differently by making the most of their situation, in whatever time they have left. By accepting that life may be shorter, they can still learn to feel empowered and begin to live life to the fullest. We often take life for granted, thinking that we can always do things in the future. Illnesses like cancer make us realize that we don't have endless time. We are all going to die. The way to live life to the fullest is to enjoy life as much as we can now.

Joe and Tammy: Problem Solving to Gain Control

Problem solving is another way to feel more in control of your life. Helplessness is reduced when you identify a problem and start to tackle it in a systematic manner. Problem solving involves the following steps:

1. Define the problem.

2. List alternative ways of coping with the problem.

3. Evaluate the various alternatives; think of the advantages and disadvantages of each alternative.

4. Select the alternative or set of alternatives with the most advantages and the least disadvantages.

5. Implement and evaluate the effectiveness of the alternative(s), and if the outcome is unsuccessful, go back to the first step and repeat the process.

Joe and Tammy are a couple who used problem solving when they were having trouble dealing with the oncologist who was treating their son. They had difficulty getting information from this physician and felt so intimidated by him that they were afraid to ask him questions. Their psychologist, Dr. David Robbins, helped them to problem solve by first defining the problem. With David's help, Joe and Tammy arrived at the following definition of the problem: "What should we do about our son's oncologist, who is reluctant to give us information?"

Joe and Tammy then moved on to brainstorming. In brainstorming, you think of alternatives that could be possible solutions to the problem. You don't evaluate the alternatives at this point, and you don't concern yourself with their advantages or disadvantages. You allow all ideas, good or bad, even wild ideas. By aiming for as many ideas as possible, you will arrive at alternatives that you might not have otherwise considered. As a result of their brainstorming with Dr. Robbins, Joe and Tammy came up with the following list of alternatives:

- We could switch to another oncologist.

- We could be more persistent with the oncologist.

- We could express our frustration to the oncologist.

- Dr. Robbins could talk to the oncologist.

- We could speak to the referring doctor.

- We could write a letter to the oncologist outlining our feelings.

- We could write a letter to the oncologist with our questions.

- We could do nothing.

After brainstorming, the next step involves eliminating the unacceptable options. In Joe and Tammy's case, they immediately eliminated the alternative of doing nothing. The next step is to evaluate each remaining alternative. The advantages and disadvantages of each alternative is discussed. As part of the evaluation, the likelihood of success of each alternative is also considered.

Joe and Tammy did a pros and cons list for each of the other alternatives. After weighing the pros- and cons- of each alternative, the parents decided that the best thing to do was to be more persistent and confront the doctor. David then taught them how to be assertive with the doctor. Through role-playing, he showed the parents how to confront the oncologist without sounding hostile. Although the oncologist wasn't particularly receptive, the parents nevertheless felt more in control in their dealings with him.

How to Use This Book

The first chapter, "Empowerment," gives you a preview of the most common problem encountered by cancer patients. The next chapter takes up the crucial issue of choosing a fighting attitude toward your cancer. Chapter 3 teaches you various ways to overcome depression; chapter 4 offers techniques to control anxiety and stress, and in chapter 5 you will learn how to cope with pain. Chapter 6 can help you work through any grief you may experience. Chapters 7 and 8 encourage and teach you to love yourself and reach out to others. You can read the book through first or look to the next section to develop your own coping plan, picking and choosing which issues you would like to approach first.

Your Personal Coping Plan

In order to help you select the appropriate strategies for specific problems, we offer you the following problem-solution outline. Look through the list of problems and use it to help identify your own. Then examine the corresponding coping strategies that you can use, referring to the chapters that describe, in detail, how to use these skills.

As you develop your own program, feel free to modify the techniques and recommendations to suit your own needs. You don't have to follow a formula—our suggestions and transcripts are intended to be guidelines, not rules.

Problem-Solution Checklist

Problem	Solution	Chapter
Anxiety	Relaxation	4
	Self-hypnosis	5
	Imagery	4
	Cognitive therapy	4
	Problem solving	1
	Desensitization	4
	Stress Innoculation	4
Depression/Guilt	Cognitive therapy	3
	Goal setting	3
	Pleasurable experiences	3
	Reaching out	8
	Assertiveness	7
Pain	Relaxation	4
	Self-hypnosis	5
	Imagery	4
	Cognitive therapy	5
	Relabeling	5
Passivity	Pleasurable experiences	3
	Goal setting	3
Isolation	Communication	8
	Assertiveness	7
	Support groups	8
	Computer networking	8
Sexual Difficulties	Cognitive therapy	8
	Communication	8
	Sex therapy	8

A Fighting Spirit: Becoming a Cancer Survivor

How often have you heard that athletes become consistent winners when they possess a fighting spirit? Coaches will often refer to good players as having an ability to persist, or fight, regardless of whether they are favored to win or lose. Underdogs are not supposed to win. However, there are plenty of examples that show underdogs are not to be taken for granted as guaranteed losers.

Just ask George Foreman who, at the age of forty-five, became the oldest man to regain a heavyweight title. Although he was expected to lose, he never gave up. When given the opportunity, he fought like a champion. George Foreman knew that what he told himself about his ability would determine whether he had a chance to win. When he was interviewed after the fight, he said that in order to win he had to ignore everyone who said he had no chance. Instead, George Foreman believed in himself. Using his own form of mind control, he psyched himself into believing he could and would win. George Foreman truly had a fighting spirit.

To win, you have to believe that you can.

At this point you may be wondering what winning in a sporting event has in common with fighting cancer. A great deal. To believe that you can fight your illness and not let the illness control you is similar to fighting any opponent, whether it be in the boxing ring or in your body. To win, you have to believe that you can. This is called the fighting spirit.

You might say that a fighting spirit is having a realistic conception of what is happening, without being defeated by this information. In other words, most people are afraid of serious illnesses such as cancer because they have only heard the horror stories about how cancer will destroy the spirit and the body. On the other hand, if you speak with people who treat the illness, you find that more people than ever before are living much longer than they would have only a few years ago. And there is medical evidence to support this:

Dr. David Spiegel (1993) and his associates report research on the benefit of committing to a support group and learning certain skills such as self-hypnosis for pain. The women in Dr. Spiegel's research study had metastatic breast cancer. It was found that the patients in the cancer support group enjoyed a better quality of life and lived twice as long as the patients who received only traditional medical treatment.

Similar results were found by Dr. Fawzy (1993) and his associates at the University of California at Los Angeles (UCLA) School of Medicine. In this study, patients with malignant melanoma received a number of therapeutic interventions, many of which are described in this book. They were taught stress management techniques and other coping skills, and received education about their illness, nutritional counseling, and supportive group counseling. The patients receiving this combination of treatments were less likely to experience a recurrence, and were less likely to die than patients who did not receive these interventions.

This is not to say that if you have a fighting spirit, you will absolutely cure your illness. But a fighting spirit will help you feel more empowered and live a more productive and happy life.

This chapter is going to teach you how to fight and remain realistic about your expectations of success. The sooner you embark

---

Accept the diagnosis but defy the prognosis.

on a program to fight your illness, the better your chances will be of feeling more in control and less like a victim. A great phrase that clearly demonstrates this concept is the one coined by Norman Cousins in his book *Head First: The Biology of Hope* (1989): "Don't deny the diagnosis, just defy the verdict that is supposed to accompany it." Another way of saying this is Accept the diagnosis but defy the prognosis.

Decide How to Fight Your Cancer

When Dr. David Robbins, our third author, was first told of his diagnosis he was depressed for several weeks. Then he realized that he had been teaching his patients how to fight cancer for many years and now it was his turn to fight. David began his battle by problem solving. He decided that he needed to gather as much information about his type of cancer as he could. Through problem solving, he determined that the best way to start this process would be to use his contacts in medicine. He called upon friends in the field for advice and support, and, with the help of this advice, was able to compile a list of top doctors. Then, he and his wife, Helene, began calling these experts for advice. They learned through these new contacts that surgery, chemotherapy, and radiation therapy were the standard procedures for this type of cancer.

David's thoughts about his illness started to change after the success of his problem solving. His newly proactive attitude helped him feel less like a victim. Where he once thought that all hope was gone, he now felt he was given renewed hope and a real chance for survival. He started to think more positively. He began to realize, "I have my wife, my two daughters, very good close friends, and so much to live for." He focused on his strengths and what he wanted to do in the future, setting goals to live for. This book is the result of one of those goals. Some of his other goals included teaching his younger daughter, Erica, how to drive, and seeing his daughter, Donna, graduate high school in two years.

Another primary objective for David was to return to work and continue counseling his patients. David felt inspired to teach his cancer patients the techniques he had found so useful for himself. Within a month after surgery he returned to work, first on a part-time basis. He then gradually increased his workload until he was able to resume working full-time. Throughout this period he remained optimistic, believing that he would survive. He truly lived with the fighting spirit.

Another dramatic demonstration of the fighting attitude occurred with a patient named Mat who was diagnosed with esophageal cancer. Mat researched his illness and read articles about the treatments and the survival rates of patients with his illness. He read that this is a very serious and deadly form of cancer. He also read that, by the time most of these cases are diagnosed, the patients have less than one year to live. It often strikes older people who have a long history of cigarette and/or alcohol abuse. In this case, Mat was a young man of only forty years who did have some history of smoking but no alcohol abuse.

When he was diagnosed, he was immediately scheduled for surgery. He had a good deal of his esophagus and part of his stomach removed. While he was in the hospital, right after surgery, he asked his surgeon what his chances of survival were. He was then informed that he should not think of signing any long-term mortgages. Of course, this was a devastating thing to be told, and it sent Mat into a depression. His surgeon obviously did not realize the negative impact of his words.

Without any guidance, Mat was uncertain what he could do. He was aware of the American Cancer Society, and he thought that maybe they could guide him. He was lucky in that they do have a crisis counseling program. This program is designed to provide patients and their families with counseling from a licensed professional. The American Cancer Society referred Mat to Dr. Wayne Gersh.

At the beginning of counseling, Mat was feeling totally hopeless and devastated. However, he seemed to sense that doing something was certainly better than doing nothing, even though all the statistics seemed to be against him.

From the beginning of counseling with Wayne, Mat was intent on fighting. He felt that with nothing to lose and everything to gain he was going to learn as much as he could about his illness and fight it. His wife was a major part of his support system, although there were times when her fear was as great as his. Unfortunately, she was not always able to hide her fears and this made it difficult for him to remain strong. Another difficulty was his job, which he didn't like, but which provided him with medical insurance. Now he felt stuck because he needed the medical insurance to help pay his expenses.

As his counseling with Wayne continued, he started to realize how much he could do to fight his illness. He could join support groups; go to workshops on medical techniques; and learn specific techniques from counseling such as relaxation, assertiveness training, and positive thinking.

One of the more impressive gains Mat made was his ability to alter his and his wife's view of his career and his future. He was able to convince himself, and eventually his wife, that he deserved to live a life that was happy and filled with experiences that he wanted. This led to his quitting his job and starting his own business even though his wife was terrified. She believed what the statistics said—that he was going to die quickly. With Wayne's help, Mat was able to convince her that her fears, though realistic, were not helpful to him. When she first came to his counseling sessions, she said, "I'm afraid that if he changes his job he'll lose his insurance. I'll be stuck with a lot of medical bills and no husband." Wayne said, "You have good reason to be afraid. Anyone in your situation would feel just as you do. Maybe we could figure out a way that Mat could leave his current job and still keep his insurance. Why don't you contact the state insurance department and find out what the rules are? Mat, have you explained what your reasons are for wanting to leave your job?" Mat replied, "I want to still have a life, regardless of how long I live. Quality of life is very important to me. I need a reason to live. This gives me something to fight for." Wayne explained that having goals and a reason to live usually results in less depression and anxiety and a better quality of life for most cancer patients. It also may improve a patient's chances of survival.

Mat and his wife researched the insurance issue and discovered that he could obtain insurance with no loss of coverage. With Wayne's ongoing help, Mat's wife was able to deal with her anxieties and continued to be a source of strength and support for her husband. Mat left his job and embarked on a new career. Four years later, he is still living and happy. When Wayne last spoke with him, Mat was positive and optimistic. "I'm so glad I left my old job. It's great to be my own boss, and I'm making more money than I did before. My wife is more secure about it too. I just know that whatever happens, I made the right decision." Mat also reported that his surgeon told him that he didn't need to be seen as frequently, due to his excellent response to treatment.

You're Not to Blame

Dr. David Spiegel, a renowned psychiatrist and hypnotherapist, has been very critical of approaches that teach patients to fight their illnesses. Although he has shown in his own research that the mind can influence bodily responses, he correctly points out that some therapeutic approaches encouraging a fighting attitude can engender guilt in those patients who are not successful in curing their illnesses. He also points out that another guilt-inducing message is that you are responsible for your illness. It is very easy to assume that if you are responsible for your illness, then you caused it. In fact, most cancer patients are not responsible for their illness. Psychological factors play little or no role in causing cancer. For every study that reported discovering the existence of a cancer-type personality, there are more studies that contradict it. Some cancers, such as lung cancer, may be caused by carcinogens such as cigarette smoking. However, you still do not have to feel guilty even if your cancer can be linked to cigarette smoking or some other unhealthy behavior. Guilt is not a constructive emotion. The way to rid yourself of all guilt is first to question whether you are, in fact, responsible. And even if you are responsible, as in the case of cigarette smoking, you can forgive yourself and focus on what you can do to maximize your chances of survival and enjoy your life as much as you can.

> Guilt is not a constructive emotion.

Keep in mind that despite Dr. Spiegel's skepticism about being able to fight cancer, he reports that patients in his cancer support groups enjoyed a better quality of life and lived longer than patients not receiving supportive group therapy. Some of the methods that were used in his support groups include self-hypnosis for pain control and encouragement to express feelings. Rather than rejecting techniques for fighting cancer, we think a more balanced approach is to include them as part of your repertoire of techniques for coping with cancer. You really have nothing to lose by using these techniques, as long as you recognize their benefits and limitations.

Abe: Overcoming Feelings of Helplessness

An interesting example of how a patient can learn to be a fighter after initially giving up is the case of Abe, who, at age sixty, was diagnosed with lung cancer. Abe was traumatized by his diagnosis and was totally unable to function. Although he was able to move around freely, he was unable to work because his job as a plumber was too strenuous. Despite his potential to enjoy most aspects of life, he acted as if his life was over and he was no longer competent at even the most basic tasks. He believed, as many patients believe, that your life is over when you are told that cancer has struck.

Abe came for counseling with Wayne. At the beginning, Abe was assessed as being highly anxious and depressed. Instead of fighting, he would act as if he couldn't engage in the simplest of tasks without his wife helping him or caring for him. When faced with appointments for counseling, Abe often tried to cancel and asked his wife Doris, to make the phone call. Doris wanted to help him, but she didn't know what she should encourage him to do on his own. She was furious with him for acting so helpless.

Wayne met with Abe and Doris, focusing on Abe's helplessness. "I know that having this illness is frightening to you. I can understand why you may want to avoid dealing with your situation. A lot of people feel like giving up at this point. However, I can help you feel less anxious and depressed. My patients do much better with counseling when they are active participants. So, I would like you to make your own appointments and come regularly." Abe reluctantly agreed.

Wayne encouraged Doris to be assertive and to prompt Abe to do more for himself. This immediately enabled Doris to assert her rights. The reason why she had difficulty being assertive with Abe was because she felt sorry for him and felt guilty if she refused any of his requests. This left her feeling resentful toward Abe because she felt trapped and burdened. Doris felt empowered by Wayne's encouragement for her to be assertive, and she told him, "I feel so relieved. I didn't know what to do. I felt so guilty saying 'no' to Abe, but I was hating doing everything for him. I feel you just gave me permission to live more like we did before."

In many cases, family members think that to help the patient, they must take full responsibility for their loved one's life. This only serves to infantilize the patient. You don't have to let this happen to you. You don't want to give up responsibility for yourself, because it only reinforces feelings of helplessness.

Abe started to respond to counseling. He gradually came to realize that he was still competent in many areas. Although he was not able to work, he was still able to be with friends, travel, and generally live a normal life. He started to take an active role in his treatment and went into remission. Yet, after several months of feeling very positive and in control, Abe had a recurrence of cancer. The illness had spread to his throat, and he reverted to acting in a helpless manner. With continued help from his wife and Wayne, Abe started to fight again. Once again his illness went into remission, and he realized that he was able to fight if he continued to believe and try. Unfortunately, Abe had another recurrence. This time the cancer had spread to his brain. It was at this point that his wife was told by his physicians that he was probably going to die within several months, but she didn't tell Abe. He, not knowing that he was supposed to die, just kept fighting. He was, at this point, a strong believer in the power of his mind to fight cancer, and he would not give in to his illness. Three relapses later, he did eventually die. However, his death occurred more than three years after his wife was told that he only had months to live. The medical personnel treating him were amazed by his resistance. It seems as though Abe's fighting spirit bolstered his immune system, which enabled his body to fight the cancer. Abe would probably have been the first to tell anyone who would listen that his desire to live kept him alive, long after others had expected him to die.

> *In many cases, family members think that*
> *to help the patient, they must take full*
> *responsibility for their loved one's life. This*
> *only serves to infantilize the patient.*

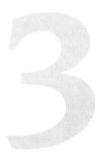

Looking Ahead
Positively

There are three different patterns of thinking that can cause you to feel depressed. They can be classified according to whether they involve self-condemnation, hopelessness and helplessness, or self-pity. Knowing how to identify your specific pattern of thinking will enable you to use the most effective strategies in fighting depression.

Some patients feel guilty because they blame themselves for having gotten cancer. Guilt is a type of depression that stems from two beliefs: that you are responsible for causing your illness, and that you are stupid, bad, or worthless for having caused it. Certain behaviors like cigarette smoking are linked to cancer, and it is therefore plausible that you contributed in some manner to your illness—but this does not mean that you should condemn yourself. It never helps to condemn yourself, even if you did engage in unhealthy behavior. Blaming yourself is never constructive. A better approach is to recognize that you are a fallible human being who makes mistakes. So forgive yourself, and let us help you figure out what you can do now to make the most of your life.

Beverly: Guilt Feelings Leading to Depression

Beverly came to counseling with Dr. Bill Golden after receiving a diagnosis of lung cancer because she wanted to learn how to stop smoking. She told Bill, "I feel so guilty about having gotten lung cancer. I've smoked ever since I was a teenager, and I know this is how I got cancer. What I would like to do is to stop smoking. I must do this—I hope it's not too late. I should have quit years ago. Boy, am I stupid!"

Bill was able to help Beverly quit smoking by teaching her to use hypnosis. In addition, he noted that her guilt was causing her to feel depressed. Bill tried to help Beverly by explaining that her guilt feelings were unproductive and damaging: "I know you feel responsible for getting cancer, but to condemn yourself is unproductive and will only make you feel more depressed. You have a right to feel good about yourself, no matter what."

Beverly found Dr. Golden's intervention helpful in reducing her guilt. She came to realize that these guilty thoughts would not help her in her battle against the disease. She was successful in quitting smoking and was significantly less depressed. Although she maintained the belief that she was responsible for causing her cancer, she no longer condemned herself. She realized lots of people from her generation made the same mistake about smoking. And what's more, she realized that people still smoke, even though it is a well-known fact that smoking is carcinogenic.

Many patients make the mistake of holding themselves responsible for having caused their cancer when their behavior had nothing to do with the disease. Some people blame themselves for eating the wrong foods, for not taking vitamins, for worrying too much, thinking too negatively, being too angry, or not being angry enough. Although there is some possibility that the above factors can affect the immune system, there is no widely accepted proof that they cause cancer. And, regardless of your actions before you had cancer, now that you've been diagnosed it is crucial that you try to abandon the self-condemnation that can lead to a damaging depression.

John: Feelings of Helplessness and Hopelessness Leading to Depression

Another type of depression involves hopelessness and helplessness, a pattern of thinking that can become self-fulfilling. The person who feels hopeless and helpless may give up and drop out of treatment. Even if you don't drop out, you decrease your chances of survival when you become pessimistic and give up on yourself. Your best tool to fight hopelessness and helplessness is positive thinking. Hope is restored when you see alternatives. You don't have to be 100 percent optimistic—all you have to do is see some possibility of hope, and then act on it. Following a positive course of action will reduce feelings of hopelessness and helplessness.

> *You don't have to be* 100 *percent optimistic—all you have to do is see some possibility of hope, and then act on it.*

When John was initially diagnosed with cancer he thought, "I have nothing to look forward to. My life is over." Previously, he was a hardworking commercial film producer, a fun-loving man who was devoted to his work, his wife, and his two daughters.

It's natural to have negative thoughts after receiving a diagnosis of cancer. However, continuing to engage in negative thinking can result in helplessness and hopelessness, which is one form of depression. John's thoughts are an example of hopelessness. After finding out he had cancer, he totally gave up. Convinced that his life was over, John stopped going to work and pursuing his hobbies. Because he thought he had nothing to look forward to, he stopped reading, exercising, and going out with friends and family. He stayed home most of the time and couldn't even be coaxed by his children to play with them. John's "give-up-itis" continued for over a year. When he reached his forty-second birthday, he woke up. He remembers thinking, "Wow, it's a year later and I'm still alive. I wasted a whole year waiting to die—enough is enough. It's time to start living again."

John regained his hope and began to think more positively. He became active again. John realized that his belief that he was hopeless was just causing him to feel more depressed and to waste whatever precious time he had left.

Bonnie: Self-pity Leading to Depression

During the months following her diagnosis, Bonnie found herself frequently thinking, "Poor me, my whole life sucks. What did I do to deserve this?" Bonnie's negative thinking is an example of self-pity. Self-pity is another type of depression that results in passivity.

Bonnie, who was an active, vibrant, thirty-two-year-old woman, became unwilling to exercise, play with her children, or go to her job as a hairdresser. Fortunately for Bonnie, her husband, Hank, and her two children, Timmy, nine years old and Cindy, eleven years old, would not allow her to continue to feel sorry for herself. Her family repeatedly reminded her through words and deeds how much they loved and appreciated her. Hank constantly reminded her of all the reasons why life was worth living. He also encouraged her to enter counseling. Bonnie's customers also would not let her withdraw into self-pity. They kept calling Bonnie, telling her how much they missed her and needed her to come back to work.

Bonnie did go into counseling. After a while, Bonnie started to realize she had a lot going for her. She eventually went back to work. She started exercising and began to enjoy life once again.

John's and Bonnie's negative thoughts were self-defeating because they resulted in withdrawal and immobility. The main cause of depression in cancer patients is negative thinking. Don't despair! There are a number of strategies specifically designed for overcoming hopelessness and helplessness, as well as self-pity and guilt.

Cognitive Therapy

Cognitive therapy has been shown to be the most effective psychological treatment for depression. In cognitive therapy, you control depression by identifying and then altering your negative thoughts. Replacing negative thoughts with positive and coping thoughts helps to reduce depression.

The first step in cognitive therapy is to identify your negative thoughts. A simple procedure for identifying and modifying your negative thoughts is the two-column method. First, divide a page in half. At the top of the page, write a brief description of the situation that is causing you to feel depressed. On the left side of

> *In cognitive therapy, you control depression by identifying and then altering your negative thoughts.*

the page, write down the negative thoughts associated with your depression. Try to remember what thoughts were going through your mind immediately before you began to feel depressed, and which thoughts seemed to replay themselves in your mind as you became more depressed. The next step is to question and reevaluate these negative thoughts and to arrive at a more constructive and positive way of thinking. Reevaluate each negative thought and list constructive and positive alternatives in the right column. The goal is to construct what are called coping thoughts or positive self-statements that will counter the depressive effects of the negative thoughts. An example of Bonnie's two-column table follows:

Situation: Diagnosis of Cancer	
Negative Thoughts	*Coping Thoughts*
1. Poor me, everything happens to me.	1. Bad stuff happens. I can deal with this. There are a lot of positive things in my life, and it's worth fighting for.
2. I'm such a jerk for feeling sorry for myself. People will think I'm such a loser for feeling sorry for myself.	2. It's only natural that I feel sorry for myself. I'm going through a rough time, so why blame myself for feeling down?

Cognitive Therapy and Self-Pity

The cognitive therapy approach to reducing self-pity involves first recognizing that you are feeling sorry for yourself. This recognition can be made more difficult by feelings of shame because many people feel that they are not supposed to feel sorry for themselves. Bonnie felt that it was socially unacceptable for her to ever engage in self-pity. Her negative thoughts were: "I'm such a jerk for feeling sorry for myself. People will think I'm such a loser for feeling sorry for myself."

As we pointed out earlier, self-pity is a natural response for someone faced with a serious illness. So, the first step in Bonnie's counseling was for her to accept herself, no matter what she was feeling. The coping thoughts that she developed for self-acceptance were: "It's only natural that I feel sorry for myself. I'm going through a rough time, so why blame myself for feeling down?" Then she was able to actively engage in fighting self-pity. The rational statements that she then developed were: "Bad stuff happens. I can deal with this. There are a lot of positive things in my life, and it's worth fighting for."

Cognitive Therapy and Guilt

Philip was feeling guilty about having gotten cancer because he believed that his diet and lifestyle were contributing factors. Philip was fifty-two years old, with a wife and two teenage children, when he received a diagnosis of colon cancer. He believed that his diet, which was filled with high-fat foods, was the main reason he got cancer. When he first went to see Dr. Wayne Gersh, he said that he felt guilty about not taking better care of himself and that he felt the cancer was entirely his fault. He said, "I know it's my fault; if only I had eaten less meat. I should have listened to all those reports I always see on television about cancer and high-fat foods. Now I'm going to die and leave my family without a father. It's all my fault."

After hearing Philip describe his feelings, Wayne realized that the two-column method would be a useful tool in reducing Philip's depression. He told Philip, "Although you might have been able to change your diet, is it true that everyone you know who ate with you and shared the same foods also got cancer?" Philip responded, "I know what you're trying to do, but I still feel that I was wrong."

Wayne then went on to tell Philip that even if he was wrong, it would be better for him to forgive himself. An effective way of dealing with guilt is to accept yourself even though you may have made a mistake. Furthermore, if he felt less guilty and depressed, he would be better able to fight his illness. Wayne told Philip about the two-column method and how this could help him eliminate or reduce his feelings of guilt. Philip was willing to try this and his two-column table looks like this:

Situation: Feeling Guilty about Having Cancer	
Negative Thoughts	*Coping Thoughts*
1. I know it's my fault. I should have eaten fewer fatty foods.	1. I don't know for sure that my diet caused my cancer. But, even if it did, it's better to forgive myself and accept myself as a fallible human being.
2. It's my fault that I'm going to die and leave my family without a father.	2. I don't know that I'm going to die. My doctor says my operation was a success. There is no proof that my diet caused the cancer.

Cognitive Therapy and Helplessness/Hopelessness

Marvin, a fifty-one-year-old engineer, felt hopeless after finding out that his first trial of chemotherapy was not sufficient in completely eradicating his cancer. The doctor told him that he was responsive to treatment but just needed more. Nevertheless, Marvin was unconvinced. He did not trust his doctor. He became progressively more depressed. Finally, his wife, June, insisted that he see a psychologist.

Dr. Bill Golden thought the two-column method was ideal for Marvin because it was consistent with his manner of thinking as an engineer. Marvin was a problem solver with everything except his cancer. Bill explained to Marvin that his feelings of hopelessness and helplessness were a result of negative thinking. Furthermore, Bill helped Marvin recognize that he had the ability to look at his situation in a more constructive manner. Together, they constructed the following two-column table:

Situation: Being Told that More Chemotherapy Is Needed

Negative Thoughts	Coping Thoughts
1. I'm hopeless. Nothing can be done. The chemotherapy is not working.	1. Some people require more chemotherapy than others. My response to treatment is still positive. There is hope— I just need more treatment.
2. The doctor is lying to me.	2. The doctor is telling me what he knows, but he can't guarantee results.

Although it may seem redundant, we will continue to emphasize the two-column method because it is easy to utilize. Most of our patients prefer its simplicity over more complicated cognitive therapy techniques and forms. We present it repeatedly so that you will become very familiar with it. Eventually it will become natural and automatic for you to identify your negative thoughts and respond to them with coping thoughts.

Goal Setting

Another way of fighting feelings of depression is through goal setting. Goal setting can involve planning your future, your week, or your day, and it can include activities such as writing a book, traveling, or volunteering at a community agency. Some of you may be reluctant about setting goals for the future because you fear you may not be around to enjoy the experience. But goal setting strengthens your will to survive. Without goals we might as well be dead. Quality of life is another important issue. Regardless of how long you may live, it is important to enjoy your life to the

Goal setting strengthens your will to survive.
Without goals we might as well be dead.

fullest while you are capable. Human beings are happiest when they have hopes, dreams, and aspirations and are striving toward them. The achievement of the goal is not as important as the striving toward it. Most people think they will be happy when they achieve some goal. However, you may discover that just the planning and working toward the goal can provide great satisfaction.

David, our co-author, has found that goal setting has been one of the most important techniques he has used in his battle against cancer. David's goals included becoming more involved with his family, getting back to work as a psychologist, living a life with less anger, laughing more, and cowriting this book. He has achieved all of these goals.

As he worked toward the goal of spending more time with his family, David started going food shopping with his wife, being more available to go over homework with his daughters, communicating more with his family, and planning more family activities. David's anger-reduction goals included being less upset in traffic and being less angry with people who break rules and fail to live up to agreements. While driving, he listens to music on his CD player and laughs at other drivers who are getting upset with traffic. David's illness gave him the perspective that there are many issues that are not worth getting upset about. He learned to laugh at many of the things that used to upset him. David has come to realize that the minor annoyances of life are not worth getting upset about.

The use of visualization or imagery is another technique that works very effectively in conjunction with goal setting. When you visualize the future and see yourself achieving goals or enjoying pleasurable experiences, feelings of hope are revived. During radiation treatments, David would visualize future activities with his children and his wife. These activities included watching his children graduate high school, watching them go through college, and seeing his wife and himself as grandparents. These visualizations made David feel very optimistic that he was going to beat his illness and be around for these events.

David also used visualization to psyche himself up for getting back to work as a psychologist and getting back to his writing. He saw himself back in his office helping patients and visualized this book being sold in bookstores. His visualizations made him feel hopeful and motivated him to accomplish these goals.

On the following pages we've offered some exercises to assist you in setting goals and creating positive visualizations for yourself. Take some time out to avail yourself of these powerful techniques to improve your mind and your quality of life.

Brainstorm to Set Your Goals

Since your cancer diagnosis, you may have abandoned some goals or put others on hold. Or perhaps your cancer has inspired you to set goals for the first time in your life. This exercise will help you set reasonable goals and develop a plan to achieve them.

Use the following exercise to brainstorm some goals in various areas of your life. Within each area, try to make your long- and short-term goals related. For example, in the "Family" area, Peter related all his goals to improving his relationship to his wife, Bea:

Long-term goal	Middle goal	Short-term goal
Family reunion for our thirtieth anniversary next year	Write honest, personal letters to kids and Bea's sister over the next three months	Go to the beach house Bea likes for her birthday, and talk honestly about future

Long-term goal (1–3 years)	Middle goal (6 months– 1 year)	Short-term goal (1–6 months)

Family

Friends

Health

Finances

Profession

Spiritual

Creative

Fun

An Action Plan for Achieving Your Goals

You can create an action plan for each goal by examining your short-term goals. Just break them down into manageable steps. To accomplish your shortest-term goal, what do you need to do by one month from now? To accomplish that, what do you need to do by two weeks from now? To get there, what should you do by next week? Tomorrow? Today?

For example, Peter figured that to get back in touch with Bea, he had to follow this sequence:

Today: Tell her I'm tired of letting my prostate cancer come between us. Apologize for being so distant and grouchy.

Tomorrow: Say I want to stop isolating myself, ask her to come with me on my next doctor's appointment. Say I've changed my mind about the beach house and want to go with her.

Next week: Ask her to spade the raised bed so we can plant potatoes and onions together. Tell her about my fears and my hopes for the future.

Next month: Go to the beach house and plan the reunion.

Don't let your official prognosis keep you from making long-term plans. The literature on cancer survival is full of stories about people who lived far longer than predicted because they wanted to finish a degree, see a child graduate or get married, design one more garden, see the Greek islands, finish building a house, complete writing a book, and so on.

Not all goals have to be so organized. If the thought of making a plan that stretches out two years into the future is just too daunting for you, then you should start small. Plan just one pleasurable activity for today or tomorrow.

If you have trouble thinking of any pleasurable experiences, use the following list for ideas. Feel free to use any that you used to enjoy or might be willing to try for the first time:

- Going for a walk in the park
- Taking a bubble bath
- Going bicycle riding in a park or on a bike path
- Getting a massage
- Visiting friends
- Floating in a pool
- Swimming in a pool or a lake
- Lying on a beach under a shady palm tree
- Playing your favorite sport

- Trying a sport you have always wanted to learn
- Watching a sports event on television
- Attending your favorite sports event
- Listening to music
- Attending a concert
- Reading a good book or magazine
- Taking a drive in the country
- Renting a video you have always wanted to see
- Going to a movie theater
- Going to a play
- Speaking to friends on the telephone
- Going out to a favorite restaurant
- Going to a museum
- Knitting or crocheting
- Gardening
- Playing with your children
- Playing board games with family or friends
- Playing with video games

Once you have completed your list of pleasurable experiences, you are ready for the next step—visualization of the items from your list. Feel free to incorporate your images of positive experiences and goals into your daydreaming. Daydreaming involves imagery, so you can imagine any scene or situation you find positive and therapeutic. If a negative daydream intrudes, just change the channel, as if you were changing the channel from a television show that was making you feel uncomfortable. Find something positive to think about. Unlike television, you can almost always find something positive in your imagination to visualize. That's how you can program your daydreams.

Imagine yourself engaging in pleasurable or constructive activities from your list. These activities can occur in the near future such as the next week, or next month, or possibly several months away.

There are a number of benefits that you may experience as a result of the visualization procedure. You may experience a positive increase in your mood and an increase in your energy level. These benefits can be very helpful, in that they can instill hope and encourage you to become more active.

You will feel even more satisfaction by actually experiencing the activities on your list. However, at first you may find it difficult to become more active. Depression and your illness can cause you to feel tired and lethargic. It is important to push yourself or allow family members and friends to push you. It may be hard for you to believe that activity will give you energy when you're feeling so tired, but it will. We know from our clinical experience, as well as numerous clinical studies, that increasing activity reduces depression and increases energy.

Pick one of your favorite activities and plan to do it today or tomorrow. Write it on your calendar or wherever you usually put reminders for appointments and important events.

While you're at the calendar, schedule something pleasurable for later in the week and a couple of treats for next week and the week after. Keep going until you have a full month of pleasure planned. Keep these appointments as faithfully as you keep your most urgent appointments.

Renee's case demonstrates the use of goal setting and scheduling pleasurable activities. Renee was a forty-two-year-old woman who was diagnosed with breast cancer. When she came to counseling with Dr. Wayne Gersh, she was depressed. She was feeling helpless and hopeless. Renee stated, "It's difficult for me to get back to my usual routine. I feel like there's no purpose to it. Why bother doing anything if I'm just going to die?"

Wayne explained to Renee that becoming more active and returning to her formerly active lifestyle would help her feel less depressed. He helped her develop goals that were easy for her to achieve. These short-term goals included making phone calls to friends, going to the cinema, and attending her children's activities, such as soccer. After several weeks, she realized the value to be found in activity. She was gradually becoming more active and less depressed. She was also able to create goals that were more future-oriented, such as remodeling her kitchen. By the time she was ready to terminate counseling, she reported that she felt like her former life was returning.

Visualization

As you will remember, David used visualization hand in hand with goal setting to improve his spirits and boost his fighting attitude. You can develop positive visualizations for yourself by imagining yourself achieving your goals or by simply imagining activities that you enjoy. To help you create imagery of pleasurable activities we've provided space below for you to brainstorm.

What Do You Enjoy?

In the space provided, jot down pleasurable activities that you enjoy or used to enjoy. Some things that you used to do might not seem like fun right now, but write them down anyway. Also include activities that you have never done but might like to try.

Managing Your Stress:
Help for Anxiety

Having cancer naturally causes a great deal of stress. Symptoms of stress can include anxiety, tension, disturbed sleep, nausea and vomiting, and even avoidance of medical procedures. Some of the most effective treatments for managing these symptoms include relaxation techniques, cognitive therapy, and imagery. This chapter will teach you some of the most powerful stress-reduction techniques available to help you reduce these symptoms and improve your quality of life.

Norman: Slowing Down to Enjoy Life

Norman was a very successful insurance salesperson. He worked long hours, often leaving early in the morning and arriving home after his family had already eaten. The weekends were often used as preparation for his job. He devoted little time to the needs of his family, thinking that work was the most important aspect of his life. When he recognized that he was having stomach and bowel problems, he sought medical treatment. Testing revealed that he had stomach cancer. At age forty-three, cancer was the last thing on Norman's mind.

Although Norman underwent surgery to remove his cancer, his surgeon revealed that the cancer had spread to other areas. Norman's prognosis was that he would have only six months to live. His wife had heard of Dr. David Robbins and felt that Norman would benefit from his help.

When Norman first came for counseling, he stated that he had only six months to live. He said that his wife and family were very concerned and wanted him to prepare for his death. He appeared highly anxious and it seemed that his life was no longer in his control. David asked, "What makes you think that you only have six months to live?" "Well, the doctor told me so," said Norman. "Although this may be true, I believe you can be less anxious and regain control over your life," replied David. Norman felt skeptical but was willing to try anything at this point. He agreed to try the techniques David offered to teach him.

David felt that Norman's behavior was indicative of a highly anxious person. He surmised that a diagnosis of cancer was not the sole cause of Norman's anxiety and therefore asked Norman about his lifestyle. Norman replied, "I get up early, go to work, and come home at the end of the day." David suspected that this simple précis was not the whole story. He asked for greater detail and Norman replied, "I guess I really don't give myself time to relax. I think about my job, my customers, and how to sell more product. I'm really not eating properly, I'm still drinking a lot of coffee, and I'm not in touch with my family until I get home, which is very late at night." "This doesn't sound like a lifestyle that will enhance the quality of your life. I believe that you would benefit from learning how to relax and spend more time with your family. If you have only six months to live, wouldn't it be better to learn how to relax and live a happier life?" asked David. Norman realized David's recommendations made sense and began to work on lifestyle changes.

> *If you have only six months to live,*
> *wouldn't it be better to learn how*
> *to relax and live a happier life?*

The program that was developed for Norman included relaxation training with imagery, cognitive therapy, and specific lifestyle changes such as reducing his coffee intake and altering his work habits. These techniques, as well as other stress-management techniques, will be described in greater detail later in this chapter. In Norman's case, he was able to reduce his workload and start to concentrate on having a better quality of life. He started to eat regularly and was home at an earlier hour so that he could spend time with his family. They went on a vacation to Bermuda. Although Norman died a year later, this was longer than his original prognosis. But more important, Norman's family agreed that his last year was one of the best that they had ever shared together.

> *Norman's family agreed that his last year was one of the best that they had ever shared together.*

As you can see from Norman's story, he suffered from a significant level of anxiety when confronted by his cancer prognosis. His uncertainty about his future produced feelings that he believed were not under his control. Norman was able to control his stress and make significant lifestyle changes as a result of the stress-management techniques he learned from David.

Illness- and Nonillness- Related Stress

Norman exhibited both illness-related stress and nonillness-related stress. Illness-related stress stems from various aspects of one's illness, such as hearing one's diagnosis or prognosis. Nonillness-related stress is the result of other events in one's life, often predating the diagnosis. Examples of nonillness-related stress include on-the-job stress, marital conflict, a demanding lifestyle, or self-imposed demands such as those stemming from perfectionism. Norman's work habits were an example of nonillness-related stress.

Illness-related stress occurs often in patients that we have seen for counseling. Norman was overwhelmed with information about his illness. He felt unable to manage the stress he experienced in response to his diagnosis and prognosis. Although he incorrectly believed that he was in control over other facets of his life, his illness was one area where he believed he lacked control. He needed to learn specific stress-management techniques to restore his feelings of control.

Norman was able to manage his stress because he recognized the need to change his behavior, in addition to learning specific stress-management techniques. As we have emphasized throughout this book, cancer is the source of a great deal of stress. Learning how to manage this stress is an important aspect of any cancer-treatment program. In addition to helping you feel better, one of the benefits of controlling stress is an increased sense of competency. When you learn specific stress-reduction techniques, you will be better able to control anxiety stemming from fear of dying and fear of pain and suffering, as well as fears of the unknown associated with cancer. Learning to cope with stress will empower you and provide you with a feeling of control over your life.

Patients who are successful in coping with cancer tend to be more positive thinkers and choose to take a more assertive and active role in their treatment. They use coping thoughts that can reduce anxiety and stress such as: "I can deal with this;" "My family will learn how to deal with this as well;" "I will take control of this illness and enjoy every day I have left;" "I will do everything I can to fight this illness."

On the other hand, people who have difficulty coping with stress tend to view their situation in a more hopeless fashion and view themselves as helpless. They do not fight or take an active role in their treatment procedures. We have seen patients who have fallen into the trap of believing that cancer is a death sentence. They become paralyzed with fear and initially refuse to engage in the simplest of behavioral changes.

Relaxation Techniques

When practicing relaxation, the room should be quiet and the lights in the room should be dim. The use of a reclining chair or comfortable couch is helpful. Alternatively, you could use your bed.

Relaxation is a skill. Learning will be gradual and, as with any skill, practice is necessary.

Relaxation is a skill. Learning will be gradual and, as with any skill, practice is necessary. We recommend that you practice the relaxation procedures at least once a day, preferably twice a day. Do not be concerned if you don't master all of the techniques. Most people find that they respond well to some of the relaxation techniques but not all of them. Use the ones that work for you.

You might experience different sensations, such as tingling or drowsiness, that are related to the relaxation process. There is nothing to fear from these sensations. You will remain in control and can open your eyes at any time, although the best results will be obtained by keeping your eyes closed while resisting unnecessary movement. But if necessary, feel free to readjust the position of your body. If you wear contact lenses, you might want to remove them so that you can keep your eyes closed without the possibility of eye irritation.

Breathing Techniques

Relaxation can be produced through slow, deep breathing. During deep breathing, also known as abdominal or diaphragmatic breathing, the abdominal area rises during inhalation and flattens during exhalation. You can check to see if you are breathing deeply by placing one hand on your abdomen and the other hand on your upper chest. If you are breathing correctly, only the abdominal area will rise. Another useful technique involves lying on a flat surface such as a couch and placing a book or box of tissues on your stomach. With abdominal breathing, the book or box of tissues will rise during inhalation and descend during exhalation.

A slow, relaxed rate of breathing is approximately eight seconds to complete a full breath, including both an inhalation and exhalation. You can check to see if you are breathing at a slow, relaxed pace by counting to four as you inhale and four as you exhale. If you can't extend your breath for a count of eight, then try a count of three seconds to inhale and three to exhale. Find a breathing rate that's comfortable for you.

Also try breathing through your nose as opposed to breathing through your mouth. Breathe in through your nose and out through your nose. The reason for this recommendation, as well as the reason to breathe more slowly and deeply, is to reduce your oxygen intake. With a reduction in oxygen through these breathing techniques, physiological relaxation will occur.

Don't be concerned if you don't breathe perfectly. You can reduce your oxygen intake by slowing your breathing down, through abdominal breathing, by breathing in and out through your nose, or a combination of these. Use as many of these methods as you can, and see what works for you. You don't have to depend exclusively on any of these breathing techniques in order to relax. We will now be presenting other relaxation methods. Experiment and see which ones work for you.

Progressive Muscle Relaxation

With progressive muscle relaxation, you learn to relax by alternately tensing and relaxing the various muscles of the body. The reason why you purposely tense a muscle and then release the tension is to learn to distinguish between tension and relaxation. Eventually, you'll learn to recognize feelings of tension and will be able to relax by letting go of the tension. Don't strain your muscles when tensing. Tense your muscles just enough to feel some tension. Then let go and feel the difference. The following transcript can either be memorized or recorded on a cassette tape for you to listen to, as you go through the exercise:

Make yourself comfortable. Your arms are at your sides, your hands open, your eyes are closed and your legs are not crossed. The exercise involves tightening your muscles, one group at a time. Then concentrating on the feeling of tension in a particular muscle group, then letting go and relaxing that muscle group.

We'll start with the feet and legs. Press your feet down flat, as if you were pushing through the floor. Your toes are pressed together. Study the feeling of tension from tightening your muscles. Hold the tension. And now, let go. Just relax. Feel the tension flow out. Let both legs hang loose and limp. Relax your toes by letting them spread apart. Feel the relaxation in your ankles, calves, and knees. Relax your thighs. Let the tension go. Feel more relaxed.

Now the muscles of your abdomen. Tighten up your abdominal muscles. Study where you feel the tension. Hold it. And now relax. Feel the tension flow out. Concentrate on the feeling of relaxation. Just let go. Feel more and more relaxed.

Now your back muscles. Arch your back and feel the tension. Feel the tension in the muscles along your spine. Feel it. Just hold it. And now, let go. Let your back go limp. Feel the relaxation spreading up and down your spine.

Now your shoulders and neck. Shrug your shoulders. Tense your shoulders by raising them, lifting them up toward your ears. Feel the tension. And now, relax your shoulders by lowering them. Find a comfortable position for them, letting them hang loose and limp. Relax your neck by finding a comfortable position for your head and neck. Feel the tension flowing out. Letting go and feeling more and more relaxed.

Now your hands and arms. Make a tight fist with each hand. Make your arms stiff and straight. Feel the tension. You feel it in your fingers, forearms, upper arms and shoulders. And now, relax. Hands open, fingers apart, arms hanging loose and limp, shoulders in a comfortable relaxed position. Feeling the relaxation spreading up and down your arms, spreading all the way down to your fingertips.

Now your facial muscles. Clench your jaw. While keeping your jaw tight, push your tongue against the back of your teeth. Also press your lips together. Feel the tension this produces in your jaw, your cheeks, and your lips. Now let go and relax. Let your jaw hang slack, teeth slightly parted, lips slightly parted, tongue in a comfortable position. Feel the relaxation in your jaw, cheeks, and lips.

Now close your eyes tight, feeling the tension around your eyes and at the bridge of your nose. Hold it, but don't strain. And now, relax. Let go of the tension at the bridge of your nose. Your eyes are closed gently. Feel the tension flowing out. Feel the relaxation. Now tense your forehead by raising your eyebrows. Feel the tension in your forehead and scalp. Now let go and relax. Lower your eyebrows and feel your forehead becoming smooth and relaxed.

Continue to let go and relax. With each exhalation, letting go more and more. Breathing slowly and deeply, becoming more and more relaxed.

Letting-Go Relaxation

The next step in learning muscle relaxation involves letting go without first having to tense the muscles. After several weeks of practicing the progressive muscle-relaxation exercise, you will become more aware of tension and be better able to let go of it. At that point, it will be fairly easy and natural for you to let go of tension without first tensing. You will then be ready to begin using the following exercise, which you can memorize or record on a cassette tape:

Find a comfortable position with your arms and legs hanging loose and limp. Your eyes are closed. Let your breathing slow down, so that

*you're breathing slowly and deeply. With each exhalation, you are letting
go of tension, one muscle group at a time.*

*Start with your feet and legs. Let your toes relax by letting them
spread apart, and feel the relaxation spreading throughout the muscles
of your feet. Let both legs hang loose and limp. Let go of any tension
in your ankles, calves, knees, and thighs. Let go with each exhalation,
feeling your legs becoming more and more relaxed.*

*Now let go of any tension in your stomach. Let your stomach
muscles relax. Continue to breathe slowly and deeply. And with each
exhalation, let go, feeling the relaxation spreading throughout the abdominal area, spreading more and more, spreading to your chest.*

*Now relax your back by letting it go limp. Sink into the chair,
couch, or bed, letting your back become loose and limp. Find a comfortable
position for your head and neck, and feel the relaxation spreading up
and down your spine.*

*Next your shoulders, hands, and arms. Find a comfortable position
for your shoulders. Let your shoulders hang loose and limp, arms hanging
loose and limp, hands open, fingers apart, wrists limp. Feel the relaxation
in your upper arms, lower arms, spreading all the way down to your
fingertips.*

*Now let your jaw hang slack in a relaxed position, teeth slightly
parted. Lips slightly parted. Feel the relaxation in your jaw, cheeks, and
lips. Let go of any tension at the bridge of your nose and feel the relaxation spreading to your forehead and the muscles around your eyes.
Continue to breathe slowly and easily, feeling yourself drifting into deeper
and deeper relaxation. Continue to relax for as long as you want.*

*When you feel ready to end the relaxation, you can start to slowly
move a little at a time, moving your fingers, your toes, your arms, your
legs. Then slowly open your eyes, feeling wide awake and alert.*

Mantra Meditation

A mantra is a pleasant sounding word such as "om," "one"
or "calm," which you repeat to yourself silently for the purpose
of achieving a relaxed state. The mantra can be used by itself or
in combination with the breathing technique described earlier. You
can meditate anywhere from two to twenty minutes. Breathe
slowly and deeply. With each exhalation repeat the mantra silently.
Don't be concerned if stray thoughts enter your mind. Just let them
pass and return to the mantra. Also, don't be concerned if you
forget to repeat the mantra. Just continue to repeat it during the
next exhalation.

Imagery

Imagery can also be extremely useful for relaxation. Relaxation imagery works best when used in combination with other relaxation techniques, so, you might start with muscle relaxation, followed by slow, deep breathing. Then you could deepen the relaxation with a pleasant image.

Here is an illustrative example of a relaxation image. To get the most out of this scene, tape-record it in a slow, soft voice so that you can play it back whenever you need to relax.

Close your eyes and imagine that you are lying on a soft, sandy beach. Hear the sound of the waves lapping on the shore. Smell the fresh, warm air with its hint of salt water. Feel the warm sun bathing every inch of your body, soaking into your muscles and making every muscle in your body soft and warm. Hear the calls of seagulls coming to you on the gentle breeze. Feel the gentle breeze caress your body, keeping you from becoming too warm.

Imagine the deep blue of the sky, the golden yellow sun, and the white puffy clouds. See the deeper blue green of the ocean at the horizon. Notice how the ocean gets lighter closer to the shore. Enjoy the stately, steady swells that flow toward the shore. Watch them build and curl and finally break, foaming up onto the sand, one after another, every one different and yet every one the same. This is the deep, steady pulse of nature that goes on and on in hypnotic rhythm.

Imagine that you are in tune with this pulse. You are calm and at peace. This is exactly where you need to be. You have nothing else to do, no obligations or worries to distract you. You can let yourself go into a deep, deep relaxation. As you enjoy the warmth and peace of the beach, you become more and more relaxed. You might even drift off to sleep for a moment. That's fine. Just let yourself unwind and relax and continue to enjoy the beach for a while longer.

If the beach isn't your favorite place, pick a different scene. Select a place where you feel calm and relaxed. It could be a walk in the woods, or a mountain image, or a garden with beautiful flowers. Usually, people pick places where they have been and have felt relaxed.

Sara: Treatment-Related Stress and Imagery

You can use these techniques to ease the anxiety stemming from the changes cancer has brought into your life. They can also be applied to unpleasant, stressful medical procedures that you need to undergo as treatment for your cancer.

As we mentioned previously in this chapter, stress management techniques are very effective in reducing treatment-related stress. For example, many patients we have seen are prone to nausea, vomiting, and anxiety when they go through chemotherapy treatments. You may be able to identify with this problem, as it is quite common. Some patients are able to avoid nausea and vomiting with use of the new antinausea medications, such as Zofran, that are given along with chemotherapy. Nevertheless, despite antinausea medications, many patients still experience nausea and vomiting. In addition, many patients experience anxiety about their medical treatments, whether or not they experience nausea. If this is your problem, then stress-management techniques will help. Specifically, the use of relaxation techniques, imagery, distraction, and coping self-statements will help reduce or eliminate nausea and anxiety. We have found that, as a result of learning stress-management procedures, our patients are able to undergo medical procedures with less fear and fewer side effects.

A striking example of this occurred with a patient by the name of Sara. When she was referred to Dr. Wayne Gersh, she was already involved with chemotherapy to combat her cancer. Unfortunately for Sara, the chemical needed was cisplatin, which is highly toxic and almost always causes severe nausea and vomiting. When she first came for counseling, Sara reported that when she had treatment she was often in the hospital for at least a week due to the severity of her reaction. She reported that she often vomited almost nonstop for an entire week.

During the initial session with Sara, Wayne determined that without counseling for her anxiety about chemotherapy Sara might refuse further chemotherapy treatment. She was anxious and fearful of the side effects. Sara was starting to feel that the treatment was worse than the illness. Wayne felt that teaching Sara relaxation and imagery skills would accomplish several important things: First, he felt that her anxiety and muscle tension would be reduced—relaxation techniques, especially diaphragmatic breathing, reduce nausea; second, with the addition of relaxation imagery, Sara would be better able to distract herself during the chemotherapy procedure. Relaxation imagery provides distraction, in addition to being an effective relaxation technique. Distraction has been found to be effective in reducing anxiety as well as nausea.

When Wayne introduced stress management to Sara, she was receptive. She realized she needed stress management for reducing her anxiety. She was really surprised to learn that stress-management techniques also have the potential for controlling nausea and vomiting, even when medication doesn't help. Nevertheless, she was open and willing to do anything that might help her cope with the side effects associated with her treatment.

Being open to new ideas and having a willingness to try different techniques is often a sign of a patient who will benefit most from the procedure being offered. You may remember that during your lifetime, when you were offered an opportunity to have new experiences, your willingness to try led to greater learning and satisfaction.

> *Being open to new ideas and having a willingness to try different techniques is often a sign of a patient who will benefit most from the procedure being offered.*

Wayne introduced Sara to several relaxation techniques, which Sara tape-recorded for use at home. She was very receptive to the letting-go technique and diaphragmatic breathing. Sara was also able to record an imagery tape that she found very relaxing. Here is an excerpt from her tape:

"I see myself lying on a chaise lounge by a beautiful pool. I'm on vacation in Arizona. It's the middle of March, so the temperature is about eighty degrees. I look up, and I see a beautiful blue sky with no clouds. I look around, and I see this big, beautiful pool. The water is very blue and the floor of the pool is opalescent. It's very striking. I can hear the sounds of people talking, children laughing, and then quiet. It's the desert, so at times there occur profound silences. It's late in the afternoon, and most people have left the pool area. I take a deep breath, and I can smell the desert—but I also smell coconut. That's my suntan lotion. I can feel the softness of the chaise lounge and the warmth of the sun's rays on my body. Combined with a slight breeze, it feels so comforting. I can still taste the sugary sweetness of the drink that I recently finished. When I lie back and close my eyes, I feel so at peace, so relaxed. It's wonderful to be alive and so good to be this relaxed. Nothing can bother me here."

As you can see, creating a pleasant, relaxing image is fairly straightforward. You can develop and record one on your own. The guidelines are simple. Just pick a favorite place that you found to be relaxing. Remember it as vividly as you can. Try to use all five senses in developing the image. However, if you have trouble with one sense, such as smell or taste, don't be concerned. An image can be effective with just one or two sensory impressions. Most people have a favorite sense. For example, some people are more visual and find it easier to imagine visually. If you are such a person, it would be easiest for you to imagine the blue water in Sara's image. On the other hand, some people are more auditory. It is easier for them to recall and imagine sounds. If you are the type of person who favors auditory imagery, as opposed to visualization, it would be easiest for you to imagine the children laughing.

It's not necessary that your relaxation image be factual or accurate, just pleasant and relaxing. We have found that developing an image is not hard; just take your time and don't be discouraged if you have trouble. The key is to use a place that you can remember vividly. However, if you do not have a favorite place, or you have trouble recalling it in detail, use your imagination to conjure up a pleasant scene. Another alternative is to use an image from a movie, postcard, travel brochure, or painting. For example, one patient used a Monet painting for his pleasant image.

Sara practiced relaxation using her tape recordings. She practiced the letting-go relaxation and diaphragmatic breathing for the next several weeks. Before her sixth session, Sara had to go to the hospital to receive her chemotherapy. When she returned to counseling, she reported, "I used the relaxation and imagery when I received my chemo. I couldn't believe the results. I had almost no vomiting and very little nausea. I didn't have to stay in the hospital the whole week, like I've had to do in the past. I just felt so much more relaxed and in control!" Wayne replied, "I knew you could do it, and I was confident that if you practiced and believed in the process, it would work for you. Just keep using the relaxation techniques during your future treatments. It's important for you to continue to practice relaxation on a daily basis, and not just for treatment purposes. Regular practice will reinforce your relaxation skills, so you will be more likely to use it whenever you are in need of stress control."

Sara terminated treatment feeling very successful, but most important, with a newfound sense of control over her illness and her life. Sara's response to treatment is not unusual—over the years we have found that most of our patients are able to use relaxation and other stress-management techniques to manage the distress associated with medical procedures.

> *Regular practice will reinforce your relaxation skills, so you will be more likely to use it whenever you are in need of stress control.*

As mentioned in Sara's case, distraction is a component in relaxation imagery. Distraction has been found to be effective in reducing anxiety as well as chemotherapy side effects. There are other methods of distraction that can produce similar benefits. Any type of imagery can be used for distraction. You can use daydreams for distraction. You can think about your family, your job, your hobbies, other recreational pursuits, a problem you are trying to solve, or the vacation you want to go on. In addition, listening to music, playing video games, reading a book, watching television, playing board games, and talking with a friend or loved one are other forms of distraction.

Cognitive Therapy

In addition to using relaxation procedures, the use of cognitive-therapy techniques can be very helpful. Cognitive therapy is used to help change attitudes, beliefs, and thoughts that create excessive stress. As described in chapter 3, cognitive therapy involves identifying negative, self-defeating thoughts and attitudes, reevaluating them, and replacing them with constructive thoughts.

Joan: The Two-Column Method

For example, Joan entered counseling with Dr. Bill Golden after receiving her diagnosis of cancer. She felt that she would not be productive and that she would no longer be an asset to her company. In this case, Bill felt that the two-column cognitive-therapy technique would be useful in helping Joan change her thoughts. Joan's negative thoughts were: "I'll fail if I go back to work. I'll be a charity case. I won't be able to work as hard as before and will be a liability to the company." Bill and Joan came up with the following coping thoughts: "I know my work. I'm still capable of performing my job. My boss is not a person who would treat me like a charity case. He realizes that I'm capable. My boss knows I won't be able to work as hard, but it's okay. I'm capable, and therefore the company won't lose anything." The following table is an illustration of the two-column method that Joan used to construct her coping thoughts:

Situation: Going Back to Work after Being Ill	
Negative Thoughts	*Coping Thoughts*
1. I'll fail if I go back to work.	1. I know my work. I'm still capable of performing my job.
2. I'll be a charity case.	2. My boss is not a person who would treat me like a charity case. He realizes that I'm capable.
3. I won't be able to work as hard as before and will be a liability to the company.	3. My boss knows I won't be able to work as hard, but it's okay. I'm capable, and therefore the company won't lose anything.

When Joan recognized that her thinking was negative and self-defeating, she realized she didn't have to feel so intimidated about returning to work. After she employed cognitive therapy using the two-column method, Joan was able to return to work, feeling as if she belonged on the job regardless of her diagnosis.

Cognitive therapy can also be used to control negative thoughts about chemotherapy such as, "This drug is killing me, it's poisoning me; this chemotherapy is terrible, it's going to make me sick—I'd rather die." These negative thoughts increase one's anxiety about chemotherapy and also can intensify the side effects of nausea and vomiting. Using cognitive therapy, coping self-statements can be developed for use during chemotherapy. For example, instead of thinking, "This drug is killing me, it's poisoning me," you could think, "the chemotherapy is helping me, it's giving me life." Instead of thinking, "It's going to make me sick," you could think, "I'll use my coping tools such as relaxation and distraction techniques to control the side effects."

Relaxation and distraction techniques are most effective when you learn to use them before you begin chemotherapy. Then, you can prevent severe side effects and anxiety by applying these coping tools during your treatments. These techniques can also be effective for many patients who have already developed anxiety reactions and side effects from their cancer treatments. Some individuals experience severe reactions, not only to the chemotherapy, but also to previously neutral situations and objects. This process is called *aversive conditioning.* Chemotherapy itself is a primary cause of nausea and vomiting due to its toxicity, and nausea could occur every time you receive your treatment. Many people become anxious when anticipating these side effects. Without the benefit of coping skills or nausea-reducing medication, you could develop severe reactions that could become associated with events that lead up to the chemotherapy. Patients have become nauseated and anxious at the sight of the hospital parking lot, waiting room, or the intravenous pole.

Helen: Desensitization

For example, not only did Helen vomit after receiving chemotherapy, she started to get anxious and nauseated in response to a number of objects, such as the sight of the nightgown and suitcase that she used at the hospital. She actually vomited on several occasions just thinking about the chemotherapy and her past reactions. Helen developed a conditioned response to the suitcase and nightgown. This conditioning occurred as a result of the suitcase and nightgown becoming associated with the nausea she experienced during chemotherapy. Her reactions were so severe that she had to be hospitalized in order to receive her chemotherapy treatments. The hospital visits were still a source of terror for her because of the extent to which she suffered, even before she got to the hospital.

Helen came to counseling for help with her phobiclike response to chemotherapy. After hearing a complete list of her symptoms, Dr. Bill Golden explained to Helen that she had developed a conditioned aversive reaction to chemotherapy. Bill further explained to her that she became phobic to chemotherapy and the events leading up to it because of the conditioning process. The treatment for this problem is *desensitization*.

Desensitization is a technique where you practice controlling your anxiety and chemotherapy side effects in a gradual, step-by-step manner. First, you learn coping tools such as relaxation, distraction, and coping self-statements. Then you rank the situations and objects that upset you, from least to most distressing. Then, while in a relaxed state, you mentally rehearse coping with these distressing events.

Bill taught Helen several relaxation techniques. She learned diaphragmatic breathing, letting-go relaxation, and relaxation imagery. Helen's pleasant image was a beach in Hawaii. Helen had never gone to Hawaii but always wanted to go there. She was able to create a pleasant image based on travel brochures, postcards, and her imagination. She described her fantasy image in the following way:

"I'm lying on a beautiful, tropical Hawaiian beach. I'm on a comfortable chaise lounge, under the shade of a tall palm tree. I'm sipping on a piña colada. I can smell the pineapple in the piña colada. It's cool and refreshing. It tastes great. It's a bright, sunny day. When I look up, I can see a few pleasant, soft, pillowy clouds. It's warm out, about eighty degrees, but there's a cool ocean breeze. I can feel the gentle breeze against my skin and it's very refreshing. I can smell the fragrance of the ocean air and taste the salt air on my lips. The sand is clean, white, and fine. There are only a few people on the beach. There are a few children playing in the sand, building a statuesque sand castle. It's really pleasant to hear their giggling and sounds of joy. It reminds me of when I took my kids to the beach when they were little. I'm looking out at the horizon. I can see the waves and their white crests. These waves are fairly gentle. The sound they make as they wash on the shore is very soothing and relaxing. I listen to their hypnotic sound and I feel myself drifting off into a very relaxed state. Occasionally, I hear the sound of seagulls. I like that sound. They swoop down into the water to go fishing. I also see some pelicans flying by. I love those majestic birds. I can see people in the water, playing and swimming. I enjoy watching the teenagers splashing each other.

Out on the horizon, I can see some small sailboats, and far out, some surfers riding a wave. There's also an outrigger canoe riding the wave, heading for shore. I've always wanted to ride in one of those. I can imagine my husband and me in one of them.

"My image changes at this point. I'm in the outrigger canoe with Harold. He's wearing a Hawaiian lei around his neck. The outrigger canoe is manned by two native Hawaiian men. They are paddling vigorously to catch the wave. We've got it now. This is exciting! We're canoeing past the surfers. I feel the wind against my body. It makes me feel like I'm flying. I feel at peace with the world. I've never experienced such serenity."

Bill helped Helen come up with coping self-statements to be used during chemotherapy. Using the two-column technique, Helen was able to develop the following coping self-statements: "I am going to be okay, the chemotherapy is helping me and giving me life. I can control my feelings and create pleasant sensations through my relaxation techniques. I can also distract myself, read, and listen to my relaxation tape and my music. I can close my eyes, and tune out from my surroundings. I don't need to focus on what is going on during the chemotherapy. I'll just focus on pleasant thoughts, my wonderful beach image, and take a mental trip to Hawaii."

Bill and Helen identified various distressing situations associated with chemotherapy. These situations triggered Helen's conditioned response of anxiety and nausea. Bill and Helen then constructed a list of distressing items, called a *hierarchy*. They ranked the items from least to most disturbing. Helen's hierarchy consisted of the following items:

1. Walking into the admitting office

2. The sight of the nightgown used at the hospital

3. The suitcase used for the hospital

4. The nurse calling to make an appointment

5. The sight of the intravenous pole

6. Being in the hospital the night before receiving chemotherapy

7. The sight of the basin used for vomiting

8. Walking into the hospital room

9. Having to use the commode

10. The medical staff bringing out the chemical vials

11. Waiting in the hospital room for the treatment to begin

12. Starting the intravenous chemotherapy

13. Thinking about the possibility of getting side effects from the chemotherapy

After Helen developed relaxation skills, she proceeded with the next step in the desensitization process. This next step is to visualize each item from your hierarchy while in a deeply relaxed state. You take one item at a time, imagining the distressing situation as vividly as you can. Continue to use relaxation and your coping statements to reduce any negative feelings. Mentally rehearse coping with the situation, controlling any nausea and anxiety through distraction, coping self-statements, and relaxation procedures. You do not proceed to the next item on your hierarchy until you feel comfortable with the previous item. If you feel anxious or nauseated while imagining an item from your hierarchy, stop the visualization and focus on relaxation again. Then, when you feel relaxed and comfortable again, go back to the distressing item. Continue this procedure until you go through the entire list. The idea is to practice until you become less sensitive to those items on your hierarchy—thus the term "desensitization." Mental rehearsal, while in a relaxed state, enables you to become desensitized.

For Helen's desensitization, Bill first guided her through all of the relaxation techniques that she found helpful in producing a deeply relaxed state. Bill described, in elaborate detail, Helen's Hawaiian image. Once Helen was in a deeply relaxed state, she signaled Bill with a nod of her head to proceed with the description of the first distressing item from her hierarchy. Bill reminded Helen to use her coping self-statements, the diaphragmatic breathing, and the other relaxation techniques, to control any nausea or anxiety. Care was taken not to proceed to the next item from the hierarchy until she was feeling comfortable and in control of the preceding one. When Helen was ready to proceed to a new item, she signaled by nodding her head. This procedure continued until Helen was able to imagine every item from her hierarchy without feeling any distress. Bill explained that her feelings of comfort and control would transfer to the real-life situation through the same conditioning process that caused the problem in the first place. Just as she learned these reactions through conditioning, she was unlearning them through the desensitization procedure. In addition, the desensitization procedure also provided Helen with practice in using her coping tools. Helen was instructed to use the same coping tools during the actual chemotherapy.

Desensitization was successful in eliminating the conditioned aversive reaction and helped to reduce the severity of Helen's side effects from the chemotherapy. Helen found that the two most successful techniques for reducing nausea were the diaphragmatic breathing and the smell of pineapple from her Hawaiian relaxation image. Helen's experience is consistent with those of many other patients who have been helped with this procedure. Most people feel that diaphragmatic breathing is the most effective technique for controlling nausea. A number of other patients have also reported that imagery involving pleasant smells controls nausea for them as well. On the other hand, some patients find olfactory imagery to be ineffective, or even counterproductive.

Desensitization is extremely flexible and has wide application to other phobias, including fears about other medical procedures. Carol was experiencing panic attacks during her radiation treatment. Carol had a long history of claustrophobia and was afraid of elevators, restaurants, buses, and trains. However, she experienced a higher level of anxiety during radiation treatments than in any of the other situations. Therefore, she focused her desensitization treatment first on helping her to feel more in control in elevators, restaurants, buses, and trains. After she felt more relaxed in those situations, desensitization treatment was directed toward helping Carol cope with her radiation therapy. While in a relaxed state, Carol was asked to imagine herself undergoing each step in the radiation treatment procedure. Her desensitization was successful and enabled her to cope with the radiation therapy as well as her other fears.

Creating Your Stress Log

The first step in setting up your own desensitization program is to compile a list of stressful situations. Use the form on the following page to record the situations you find stressful, your painful feelings, your related negative thoughts, and some alternative coping thoughts that you might use to reduce your stress.

Generate about fifteen situations. If you have trouble finding enough situations, break extremely stressful events down into sev-

Stress Log			
Situation	Feeling	Negative Thoughts	Alternative Coping Thoughts

eral pieces. For example, going to the hospital for a radiation treatment could be broken down into entering the waiting room, taking
off your clothes, and undergoing the procedure itself.

The next step is to rank your situations in a hierarchy, starting with the least stressful and building up to the most stressful. You can use the following form to summarize your hierarchy.

1. _____ (least stressful)

2. _____

3. _____

4. _____

5. _____

6. _____

7. _____

8. _____

9. _____

10. _____

11. _____

12. _____

13. _____

14. _____

15. _____ (most stressful)

The items from your hierarchy can be concerning an unpleasant medical procedure, like chemotherapy, as in Helen's case. However, your hierarchy can contain items relating to any of the stressful events in your life. These items can be related to your illness, the medical procedures needed to treat your illness, or everyday stressful events. For example, Jonathan, who was recovering from Hodgkin's disease, was anxious about looking for a new job. He had lost his prior job as a result of his illness. His hierarchy

> *Your hierarchy can contain items relating to*
> *any of the stressful events in your life.*

was related to the stressful events associated with looking for a new job. The following is the hierarchy Jonathan developed:

1. Buying a newspaper

2. Checking help-wanted ads

3. Preparing a resume

4. Mailing a resume

5. Visiting an employment office

6. Telephoning and answering ads

7. Filling out job applications

8. Asking for references

9. Thinking about going for a job interview

10. The night before an interview

11. The morning of an interview

12. Waiting to be interviewed

13. Walking into the interview

14. The beginning of an interview

15. Being asked questions about my health

Before beginning the actual desensitization procedure, make sure that you are proficient at achieving relaxation. Use whatever techniques work for you. Experiment with the various relaxation techniques described throughout this chapter. Think about what other coping techniques you can use for a given situation. Helen, for example, used reading and music for distraction during her chemotherapy. Consider the use of coping self-statements as an additional tool. For instance, Jonathan was afraid that a prospective employer would reject him because he had cancer, so he used the following coping self-statements to control his fear about health-related questions during an interview:

"They probably won't ask me about my health. If they ask me why I lost my last job, I could tell the truth and explain that I have recovered from my illness. I'm assuming rejection, but they may be sympathetic. I don't have to be ashamed that I had cancer. I wouldn't want to work for anybody who was prejudiced against cancer patients. Sooner or later, I will get a job. I didn't deserve to get fired—I'm a good worker and have good credentials. I also have good references from previous jobs."

You can develop coping self-statements by using the two-column method or your stress log. As described earlier, first you identify and list your negative self-defeating thoughts. Again, your stress diary can be helpful for logging negative thoughts that cause excessive stress. Then develop coping thoughts to counter your negative thoughts.

After you develop your coping skills you are ready to proceed with the desensitization procedure. Go through the procedure in a quiet room, with no distractions or interruptions. Limit yourself to three or four stressful items in the hierarchy during any given session. You can tape-record the relaxation instructions and descriptions of the hierarchy items prior to the session. During a session, you may listen to such a tape or instruct yourself from memory.

Allow whatever time you need to get into a comfortable, relaxed state. After you have achieved a state of deep relaxation, imagine the first item of the hierarchy. If you should feel upset while imagining the item, use this as an opportunity to practice relaxation and coping self-statements for reducing any of your negative feelings. When you feel comfortable with that item, stop imagining it and focus on relaxation. Feel free to concentrate on diaphragmatic breathing while repeating your mantra (such as the word "calm"), or reintroduce your pleasant, relaxing image. Repeat the visualization of the same stressful item two or three more times until you feel confident that you can cope with that situation. Then, you can go on to the next item of the hierarchy. When you have the opportunity, practice the same techniques in the real-life situation.

Rochelle: Stress Inoculation

Anxiety surrounding insertion of intravenous needles is another fear we often see with our patients. Additionally, after many chemotherapy trials, patients' veins are often hard to find and access. This occurs because repeated use of veins for intravenous use can cause them to collapse and not be useful for further treatment. This problem can also create anxiety and fear.

With the use of relaxation and imagery, we have helped many patients reduce these fears and become more amenable to treatment. An interesting case was that of Rochelle, who feared needles so much that she would have a massive anxiety attack before every chemotherapy treatment. Her physician had to spend ten to fifteen minutes helping her to accept the needle. She would still cry and feel anxious throughout the entire treatment procedure, which often lasted one to two hours. Her physician referred Rochelle to Dr. David Robbins for her to learn to cope with her fear of needles.

When Rochelle came to counseling, she reported, "I'm anxious for several days before I have treatment, and I don't know what to do. It's getting to the point where I'm upset during the entire treatment. I feel that this is not good for me. I'm spending too much time and energy on fearing my treatment and not devoting enough energy to living."

In order to alleviate Rochelle's anxiety, David used a procedure called *stress inoculation.* Stress inoculation is similar to desensitization in that both procedures use relaxation and mental rehearsal. In both procedures, patients imagine themselves coping with stressful situations. Another similarity is that patients may use coping self-statements, in addition to relaxation procedures, for reducing negative feelings. The difference is that in stress inoculation, a ranked hierarchy is not used. The advantage of not using a hierarchy is that it is less time-consuming and therefore may produce more rapid results. However, with multiple stressful situations, and with conditioned aversive reactions to chemotherapy, a ranked hierarchy is more effective.

As the name "stress inoculation" implies, patients are taught how to inoculate themselves, much like taking a vaccine to avoid illness—but in this case they are protecting themselves against future stressors. In stress inoculation training, coping imagery is used. While in the relaxed state, you imagine yourself successfully coping with the stressful situation. Coping imagery is realistic. In situations such as receiving injections or other unpleasant medical procedures, you usually experience some degree of stress. Using coping imagery, you imagine that, at first, you experience distress. But instead of becoming overwhelmed, you cope with the distress and reduce your discomfort to a manageable level.

For Rochelle, this meant that she would imagine the nurse inserting the intravenous needle. First feeling anxious, Rochelle would then calm herself down, using the relaxation techniques and coping self-statements that David had taught her. Rochelle's coping self-statements were, "I can do this. The needle stick is only a momentary feeling of discomfort and I am strong enough to handle it. I want the chemotherapy. It's life-giving, and any discomfort is minimal compared to the strength of my desire to live." The therapeutic goal was for her to reduce the distress associated with needles to a manageable level. Rochelle knew it would be unrealistic to feel totally relaxed about needles.

When Rochelle was first introduced to the stress inoculation procedure, she was uncertain about its ability to work for her. She persevered and realized after a few weeks that her anticipatory fear of the chemotherapy was reduced. With continued practice, Rochelle was able to accept future treatments without the intense fear she had previously felt. She was no longer consumed by fear and anxiety. Rochelle was able to enjoy those weeks when she did not have chemotherapy, and felt more comfortable when she did have treatment.

Summary of the Rules for Stress Inoculation

Here is a summary of the rules for stress inoculation to help you remember each step.

1. Learn progressive muscle relaxation or another relaxation exercise so that you can become very calm and relaxed.

2. Choose an upcoming stressful situation that you will have to cope with.

3. Write down three or four coping thoughts that can help you get through the situation. (I can handle this . . . just relax and breathe . . . it will be over soon.)

4. Practice your relaxation technique until you are very relaxed.

5. Begin imagining the stressful situation from the beginning.

6. See yourself as having a little trouble coping, then say your coping statements to yourself.

7. Imagine that you cope successfully with the situation.

8. Repeat these steps two or three times before you actually encounter the stressful situation in real life.

You do not have to suffer with excessive anxiety and needless stress. You do not have to be intimidated by your medical procedures, nor is there any reason for you to have to discontinue them because of stress. Use the techniques from this chapter to manage and reduce your stress and anxiety. It is unrealistic for you to completely eliminate stress or anxiety from your life, especially if you are confronted with a life-threatening illness and experience invasive medical procedures. The goal of this chapter has been to provide you with the means to cope with the stress associated with your illness and your medical procedures. Remember, it takes time to develop skill in using these techniques. Be patient and persistent. You will feel more in control of your life as you develop more control over your stress.

5

Managing Your Pain

Although you may not be able to totally eliminate your pain, pain can usually be managed. With appropriate amounts of medication, pain control can be achieved. The techniques we will describe in this chapter are not replacements for medication. They are adjuncts to be used along with other pain control techniques.

Some of the psychological interventions for pain control require the assistance of a trained professional. Nevertheless, the methods that we will describe in this chapter can be employed by you alone.

The preceding chapter contains stress management techniques that can be used for pain control. Relaxation techniques and distraction can be used by you to reduce acute pain, especially when it is exacerbated by anxiety. Often there is a vicious cycle of anxiety from anticipating pain causing more pain, which then causes more anxiety. Part of the effectiveness of stress-management techniques in reducing pain occurs because any anxiety-reduction technique will break this vicious cycle.

The pain control methods that we will be describing in this chapter include self-hypnosis, which is similar to relaxation techniques but is different in some ways. Hypnosis has been found to have unique benefits in controlling pain above and beyond relaxation. These special contributions will be described later when we talk about how to utilize self-hypnosis. Some of the other pain control techniques include cognitive therapy, distraction, and activity therapy.

Types of Cancer Pain

Before we teach you about pain control methods, first let us define the different types of cancer pain.

Cancer pain is complex. It can involve physical, perceptual, cognitive, emotional, behavioral, environmental, and interpersonal factors. It is therefore very important for you to understand and evaluate your pain. First, cancer pain can be subdivided on the basis of whether it is *chronic* versus *acute* and *disease-related* versus *treatment-related*.

> Cancer pain is complex. It can involve physical, perceptual, cognitive, emotional, behavioral, environmental, and interpersonal factors.

Acute pain is intense and short term, usually of less than six months duration. It is almost always accompanied by anxiety. The distress associated with acute pain involves increased heart rate, sweating, muscle tension, elevated blood pressure, and an increased breathing rate. Most acute pain occurs prior to surgery or from invasive medical procedures such as surgery. Surgery is an example of *treatment-related pain*. Presurgical pain is *illness-related*. An example of presurgical pain is that of cancerous tumors that have grown to the point where they compress against nerves or infiltrate bone, nerve, or soft tissue. Stress-management procedures and hypnosis are often effective with acute pain.

Pain is considered *chronic* when it persists for longer than six months. Patients with chronic pain are frequently depressed and often suffer from sleep disorders and loss of appetite. They are likely to be experiencing lifestyle changes where the pain affects work performance, recreation, and social activities. Chronic pain may be intermittent, persistent, or progressive.

Intermittent pain is similar to acute pain in that it is time-limited. However, intermittent pain is chronic in that it occurs over and over. Although varying in intensity, *persistent pain* is present most of the time. As mentioned previously, depression may be a contributing factor in persistent pain.

Chronic *progressive pain* is often associated with metastatic cancer. The pain can become progressively more intense, frequent, and physically debilitating. Any and all pain relief measures should be utilized to control progressive pain. Very often patients with chronic and progressive pain are undermedicated. Some physicians are overly concerned that their patients may become addicted to or overdose on pain medication. If you are in this situation, you need to be assertive with your physician. Ask for the pain relief that you need.

There may be payoffs in intermittent and persistent pain. Payoffs are subtle benefits derived from suffering that actually, in the long run, make the pain worse. This may sound very strange, that there could be any benefit to your suffering, but we have seen many cases where these payoffs occur. For example, payoffs can include being excused from responsibilities that you are capable of performing, or receiving inordinate amounts of attention from others. These payoffs are destructive when they reinforce dependency and helplessness. In some cases, payoffs have even been responsible for increasing and prolonging pain. This can occur when payoffs lead to passivity. Being passive adds to pain. Being active reduces pain. Of course, you need to know and accept when you are truly in need of help from others. Although it can be hard to judge your limits, try to be aware of what you can and cannot do. Accept yourself with your limits. Try to maintain as normal a routine as possible. This will reduce your depression and pain. When you discover a limitation, ask for help. That's appropriate and is not a payoff for pain.

A number of factors are involved in the experience of pain. Pain is not just a physiological phenomenon. As mentioned earlier, pain can involve perceptual, cognitive, emotional, behavioral, interpersonal, and environmental factors. Think about which of these factors may be involved in your pain. Once you identify the various contributing factors operating in your situation, you will be in a position to use relevant interventions that we will be describing. For example, payoffs are often interpersonal. If you have family members who are infantilizing you, encouraging you to lie in bed and just rest, ask yourself some of the following questions: "Am I capable of doing more? Can I do this by myself or do I really need help? Might I feel better if I were more active?" If you think you can do more and might feel better doing more, be assertive with your family. Don't give in to the temporary comfort of being passive and dependent when you can do more.

According to the International Association for the Study of Pain, pain involves unpleasant sensations "associated with actual or potential tissue damage" (1979). However, a purely physical explanation of pain fails to account for phantom pain (when pain is felt in a missing limb) and fails to explain why people react differently to the same types of pain. It also fails to explain why hypnosis, acupuncture, and electrical stimulation can reduce pain.

The perception of pain is greatly influenced by attention. Many patients with chronic pain become passive and focus on their pain. The more you focus on your pain, the more pain you will experience. Distracting your attention away from pain will lessen it and, in some cases, will result in a temporary elimination of pain. Relaxation techniques and hypnotic interventions are effective in reducing pain, partly because they involve distraction. Distraction from pain can also be accomplished by listening to music, watching movies, playing with video games, or engaging in other tasks. Distraction also occurs when you maintain a normal routine and stay active.

In general, activity reduces most types of pain. There are several possible explanations as to why activity has this effect. When you are occupied, your attention is diverted away from your pain. Activity also reduces anxiety and depression, and may therefore break the vicious cycles involving anxiety, depression, and pain. Physical activity, such as exercise, may have the additional benefit of stimulating the production of endorphins, the body's natural pain reducers.

We have seen many instances when increasing the activity level of our patients was particularly effective in reducing pain and depression. However, there are a number of cancer patients for whom physical activity is not advisable. Some cancer patients experience pain only when they are physically active. Furthermore, exercise may even be dangerous if you have metastatic bone cancer. Physical activity could fracture your already compromised bones. Be careful and consider more passive types of activity such as reading, watching movies, and listening to music.

Martin: Cognitive Therapy and Pain

Pain is also influenced by your thinking. The way you perceive pain will determine its intensity. If you "catastrophize" about your pain, you will make it worse. Catastrophizing involves focusing on the pain and exaggerating it. Research has shown that one of the best predictors of success in pain management is whether or not an individual catastrophizes about the pain. Catastrophizing interferes with your ability to use coping strategies for pain control.

Cognitive therapy can be used to control catastrophic thinking. First, you identify your negative thoughts that might be increasing your pain and anxiety. Then, as we have described in previous chapters, you construct coping thoughts that you can use for reducing pain and anxiety. The two-column method can be used for this purpose.

Martin, who suffered from chronic pain as a result of metastatic bone cancer benefited from a combination of cognitive therapy, relaxation, and hypnosis. At first, relaxation and hypnosis were impossible to implement because Martin repeatedly opened his eyes, was restless, and grimaced throughout the procedures. Attempts to employ other pain control techniques such as distraction also failed. Dr. Bill Golden helped Martin to realize that he focused on the pain and catastrophized instead of concentrating on the therapeutic instructions. Several self-defeating thought patterns were identified: "Nothing is going to work. Why bother? The pain is too intense. If medication didn't help, this psycho-crap certainly won't. I'm such a coward. I should be able to stand this pain, but it's unbearable."

Bill took special care to be empathic so Martin would not think he was being criticized. After Bill helped Martin to identify his self-defeating thoughts, he said to Martin, "You're experiencing a great deal of pain and you're being too hard on yourself. Most people would have trouble coping with this type of pain. It's no wonder that you're having trouble keeping your mind focused on the relaxation techniques. But maybe we can do something about it. We might not be able to eliminate the pain but maybe you can get at least some relief."

Martin was skeptical. "How? It seems so hopeless," he said. Bill replied, "I understand why you feel that way. We've tried a lot of different techniques and so far none have helped. But it seems to me that the main problem is that the pain keeps distracting you." "Right," said Martin facetiously.

Bill persisted. "Sometimes what helps when the pain is that bad is to use what we call coping self-statements. They don't necessarily reduce the pain, but they can make it easier to handle. Would you like me to show you what I mean?" Martin reluctantly agreed, "Yeah, I guess I have nothing to lose."

Bill wrote Martin's negative thoughts in the left column of a paper folded in half. He and Martin then proceeded to construct Martin's coping self-statements. The following is the two-column method that Martin and Bill were able to eventually complete:

Situation: The Pain Becomes Increasingly Worse

Negative Thoughts	Coping Thoughts
1. Nothing is going to work. Why bother?	1. Keep trying.
2. The pain is too intense.	2. Just reduce it to a manageable level. Use brief relaxation such as slow deep breathing and think "calm" or use some pleasant imagery.
3. If medication didn't help, this psycho-crap certainly won't.	3. This can work. Let's see what works.
4. I'm such a coward. I should be able to stand this pain.	4. I'm not a coward. This type of pain is difficult to cope with.
5. It's unbearable.	5. It's intense, but I can be strong. I've survived. I can cope with it.

Bill helped Martin to arrive at coping self-statements by ex-plaining: "Thoughts such as 'nothing is going to work, why bother' are what we call self-fulfilling prophecies. I know it feels like it's true. That's understandable. You've tried a lot and so far nothing has helped. But, let's see if we can come up with a more construc-tive way of looking at the situation. Can you think of a different way of looking at it, or would you like me to make a suggestion?"

Martin came up with an idea. "What about 'keep trying'?" Bill responded, "That sounds fine. The important thing is to coun-teract the negative thought with a more constructive one. Let's try another one. The next one on your list is 'the pain is too intense.' I have a few suggestions for this one. We find that with intense pain the more you focus on how intense it is, the more intense it becomes. The best strategy is to focus on something other than the pain. But don't expect to eliminate it. That might be unrealistic. A more realistic goal is to reduce it to a more manageable level."

At this point Martin was a little more responsive. "Sometimes those distraction methods you taught me did reduce the pain a little, but I thought it should have been more." Bill explained, "Maybe a combination of techniques will work better. How about reminding yourself to just reduce it to a manageable level and use some slow, deep breathing and distraction, like thinking about something else other than the pain?" Martin responded, "Yeah, I have nothing to lose."

Bill further explained, "The idea is, whenever you catch yourself thinking a negative thought, replace the negative thought with a coping thought. Then use the other techniques, such as the deep breathing and distraction. And keep in mind they may not reduce the pain each and every time. Use them to reduce the pain as much as possible, and even when they don't reduce pain you can still use them to cope with it better."

Martin and Bill proceeded with the two-column method until they created a full set of coping self-statements. Martin combined the coping self-statements with some brief relaxation including deep breathing, along with the word "calm" and various pleasant and distracting images. Martin did experience some pain relief, despite the progression of his illness. According to Martin, what was most helpful was learning not to focus and dwell on how bad the pain felt.

Nathan: Relabeling

Another cognitive therapy technique is called relabeling because the meaning of the pain is changed by your relabeling it. For example, cognitive relabeling was used to help Nathan who had received surgery for colon cancer. Cognitive relabeling helped Nathan feel less anxious about his postsurgical pain because it helped him to perceive it as less threatening. Nathan was not seeking pain reduction. He didn't feel the need to actually reduce the sensations of pain because they were tolerable on the physical level. What Nathan found disturbing about the pain was his interpretation of it. He was extremely anxious about the pain because he thought that it indicated that his illness was progressing.

Nathan came to Dr. Wayne Gersh for counseling. Nathan interpreted his postsurgical pain as "a sign of impending death."

Wayne acknowledged that he had good reason to be anxious if the pain were life-threatening, but suggested that Nathan check with his physician to see if his interpretation was correct. Wayne told Nathan that there were interventions that could help him with his pain as well as his anxiety, but the first step was to get a proper medical diagnosis.

Nathan came back the next week reporting that his physician assured him that the pain was not life-threatening and was simply postsurgical pain. His anxiety and some of his pain were reduced when, following Wayne's advice, he relabeled the pain as "part of the recovery process from surgery."

When you use cognitive relabeling, your interpretation of the pain is the focus of change. First, identify what meaning you are giving to the pain. Are you assuming it's a sign of impending death, as in the case of Nathan? Are you assuming that you are having a recurrence? Are you interpreting the pain as a sign of your illness progressing? Of course, pain can be a warning sign and always should be diagnosed by a physician. Even changes in your condition such as increased intensity of pain or prolonged duration should be brought to the attention of your physician. However, once your pain has been diagnosed, you are free to use cognitive relabeling in order to view your pain in a less threatening manner.

> *When you use cognitive relabeling, your interpretation of the pain is the focus of change.*

Be creative and see if you can take the same pain and view it differently. For example, once you've been assured by your physician that you are not having a recurrence, relabel the pain as "simply a common annoyance that often remains from an old illness, even when you have recovered." Find a more benign interpretation of the pain that will cause you less anxiety. The pain will be the same but your benign interpretation of it will make it less threatening and therefore less anxiety-producing. Remember, as we've said before, when you reduce your fear of the pain, you will experience less anxiety and perhaps less pain. Now we will turn to hypnotic interventions for controlling pain.

Hypnosis to Control Pain

Hypnosis has been found to be effective in reducing cancer pain and helping patients cope with painful medical procedures. If you would like to review the research and clinical studies demonstrating the effectiveness of hypnosis in controlling pain, consult our textbook, *Psychological Treatment of Cancer Patients: A Cognitive-Behavioral Approach* (1992). In addition to pain control, hypnosis can provide many other benefits. It can be used for improving sleep and appetite, and has some success in helping patients with habit control, such as smoking. You can also use hypnosis for controlling anxiety and overcoming phobias. All of the stress-management techniques in chapter 4 can be used with hypnosis. For example, hypnosis can be used in desensitization and was used by the originator of the desensitization technique, Dr. Joseph Wolpe. Hypnosis has also been effective in controlling chemotherapy side effects.

Essentially, hypnosis and relaxation procedures are interchangeable. Imagery can be used while in a relaxed state or a hypnotic state. Then, why would you use hypnosis? Some people find that imagery is more vivid with hypnosis. Some people are able to achieve deeper relaxation through hypnosis. Furthermore, hypnosis has unique value in controlling pain. On the other hand, some individuals prefer to use relaxation instead of hypnosis. Use what works for you and what you feel comfortable using. Before using hypnosis, make sure you have had a proper medical diagnosis of your pain.

Countering Myths about Hypnosis

What is hypnosis? Because of the impact of the media on our lives today, most people are both informed and misinformed about hypnosis. Here is a list of statements that will help you to evaluate your own level of understanding and to clarify any misconceptions that you might have about hypnosis. Think about whether these statements are true or false:

1. Hypnosis is sleep.

2. You might not wake up from hypnosis.

3. Hypnosis weakens you.

4. Only gullible people respond to hypnosis.

5. Only unintelligent people respond to hypnosis.

6. Only emotionally disturbed people respond to hypnosis.

7. Self-hypnosis is dangerous.

All of the above statements are misconceptions about hypnosis. In order to provide you with a better understanding of hypnosis, each of these myths will be discussed. Then you will be better able to make a rational decision about whether or not you want to employ hypnosis.

People often expect or fear that they would be unconscious if they were to experience hypnosis. In fact, contrary to this notion, hypnosis is not sleep—you are not unconscious. Usually, people undergoing hypnosis report feeling relaxed. Experiments in which physiological responses are measured show that people in a hypnotic state show signs of relaxation, not sleep.

Because hypnosis is not sleep, one does not have to worry about waking up. Even if you experience drowsiness as part of hypnosis, you are not unconscious. It is possible to fall asleep during hypnosis. Falling asleep during hypnosis is like falling asleep watching television. As you know, if you fall asleep while watching television, you eventually wake up.

Hypnosis does not weaken you. Quite the opposite is true— hypnosis will help you develop greater control. Hypnosis has been used to help people stop smoking and develop control over other habits. In addition, hypnosis can help you overcome fears and phobias and give you courage to undergo invasive medical procedures.

> *Hypnosis can help you overcome fears and phobias and give you courage to undergo invasive medical procedures.*

It is untrue that only gullible people respond to hypnosis. Researchers have failed to find any relationship between hypnotic responsiveness and any negative personality traits. Research also has disproved the misconception that only unintelligent people respond to hypnosis. Actually, the opposite is true. Hypnosis requires a certain degree of concentration and intelligence. Intelligent and creative people tend to be the best hypnotic subjects. It is also untrue that if you respond to hypnosis, it means that you are emotionally disturbed. Almost everyone can learn to use hypnosis and benefit from it.

Self-hypnosis is not dangerous, it is safe to use. It is simply a state of relaxation. During the relaxed state, you will be giving yourself positive suggestions that will help you to cope with and control pain. Therapeutic effects are produced through the use of imagery and suggestion. Later, we will be describing hypnotic strategies that utilize imagery and positive suggestion for therapeutic purposes.

There are a few precautions to consider when employing self-hypnosis. As mentioned earlier, one of the few dangers of hypnosis or self-hypnosis occurs if you remove physical pain without understanding what is causing it. Before you attempt to eliminate any pain, consult your physician to get a proper diagnosis.

Another concern is whether it is possible to slip into hypnosis when it would be dangerous, such as while driving a car. Experiences similar to hypnosis are very common and are safe. They occur whenever you become so deeply absorbed in daydreaming, reading, or watching a movie that you are less aware of your surroundings.

Drivers frequently experience hypnotic-like phenomena. Did you ever have the experience of driving your car and suddenly finding yourself at your destination, without having been conscious of all the details of how you got there? This often happens to drivers when they are traveling on a familiar route. Some have said that it feels like their car is on "automatic pilot."

When on automatic pilot, you are not unconscious, nor are you totally unaware of your surroundings. When you have to stop for a red light or if there is an emergency, you're able to refocus your attention and respond appropriately. Nevertheless, we would recommend that you do not listen to tape recordings of hypnosis or relaxation while driving. They could make you drowsy and inattentive.

There are four stages in self-hypnosis:

1. Inducing hypnosis

2. Deepening hypnosis

3. Utilizing hypnosis

4. Terminating hypnosis

The first step is to use a hypnotic-induction procedure for producing a pleasant, relaxed state. We will describe three of these hypnotic-induction procedures. We will also provide you with transcripts that you can either memorize or record on cassette tapes for your personal use.

The second step involves the deepening of hypnosis. Once you have induced a relaxed hypnotic state, you may proceed to deepen it through further suggestion. The deepening of hypnosis allows for a more complete relaxation. We will describe several deepening techniques and will provide transcripts of them.

The third step is the utilization of hypnosis. During hypnosis, you can give yourself constructive suggestions, modify negative thinking, and employ pain-reducing strategies. During this stage you can also give yourself suggestions for help with other problems, such as chemotherapy side effects. In this chapter we will be teaching you hypnotic pain control strategies.

The fourth step is the termination of hypnosis. Before you terminate hypnosis, remember to remove any suggestions that you do not want remaining after your self-hypnosis session. For example, we will be teaching you a deepening technique where you make your body feel heavy, which for many people, is associated with deep relaxation. However, you may not want to walk around with that feeling of heaviness. Hypnotic suggestions can remain after termination of the hypnotic state. So, in the example of heaviness, remember to reverse the suggestion by saying, "Now my body will return to its normal feeling of weight." Don't reverse the feelings and suggestions that you want to retain after termination of your hypnosis. Posthypnotic suggestions are therapeutic suggestions that you give yourself during hypnosis that remain after termination of the hypnotic state.

You may terminate hypnosis through suggestions such as, "I will now open my eyes feeling wonderful—relaxed, refreshed, wide awake, and alert." The counting method is another approach. You count forward to a specific number, such as from one to five or ten. Suggest that, at the end of the count, you will be fully alert.

Hypnotic Induction

Hypnotic-induction procedures are very similar to the relaxation procedures described in chapter 4. There are several ways to learn how to induce self-hypnosis. You could make a tape recording of the transcripts that we will be providing you in this chapter. Some people like to use the sound of their own voice, while other people prefer to have someone else make the recording for them.

Another alternative is to memorize a transcript and repeat it to yourself silently. And you don't have to follow our script; you can also take the basic principles of hypnotic induction and apply them on your own, using your own wording. With any self-hypnotic method, you can refer to yourself in the first person as "I" or refer to yourself as "you." You can say either "I feel relaxed" or "You feel relaxed." Before starting your hypnotic induction, find a quiet place, get into a comfortable position, and close your eyes. You can use one of the hypnotic-induction procedures that we will now describe.

One hypnotic-induction procedure consists of relaxation techniques, similar to those described in chapter 4. You can use various relaxation techniques, such as slow, deep breathing, progressive relaxation, and a pleasant, relaxing image to achieve a relaxed hypnotic state. The following procedure can be modified to be consistent with your personal preferences. For example, you can refer to yourself as "I" or "you." Use a relaxation image that you have constructed.

Close your eyes and find a comfortable relaxed position. Let your breathing start to slow down so that you are breathing slowly and deeply—a comfortable, relaxed breathing pattern. You are breathing in slowly and breathing out slowly—a comfortable, rhythmic breathing pattern.

As you continue to breathe slowly and deeply, your whole body will become relaxed, starting with your arms and legs. Your arms and legs are starting to relax. Arms and legs hanging loose and limp, just as if you were a rag doll. Hands open, fingers apart, wrists loose and limp. Feel the relaxation spreading up and down your arms, all the way up to your shoulders. Let your shoulders hang comfortably. Feel the relaxation spreading.

Your legs are hanging loose and limp. Feel the relaxation spreading all the way down to your toes. Feel your toes and feet relax as you let your toes spread apart. Feel the relaxation in your ankles, calves, knees, and thighs. Both legs becoming more and more relaxed.

Notice that with each exhalation you can feel yourself becoming more relaxed. Feel the relaxation spreading with each exhalation. Breathe slowly and deeply. With each exhalation feel yourself sinking into a deeper relaxation.

Feel the relaxation spreading to your back and neck. Let your back go loose and limp. Feel the relaxation spreading to your neck. Let your jaw hang slack, teeth slightly parted. Feel the relaxation in your jaw and lips. Feel the relaxation spreading to your facial muscles. Feel the relaxation spreading to your cheeks, your forehead, the muscles surrounding your eyes.

Feel the relaxation spreading throughout your body, permeating your body. Continue to breathe slowly and deeply, feeling more and more relaxed.

To deepen your relaxation, you can imagine your peaceful, relaxing scene. Imagine it as clearly and as vividly as you can: What it looks like . . . what you would see if you were there now . . . what you would hear . . . what you would feel . . . what you would smell. . . . Perhaps you can even use your sense of taste. . . . Keep on imagining your peaceful scene. Continue to breathe slowly and deeply. Feel yourself becoming more and more relaxed. As you continue to imagine your peaceful, serene scene and continue to breathe slowly and deeply, you become more and more relaxed.

Another method of hypnotic induction is the eye-fixation technique. Pick a spot and keep on staring at it until your eyes get tired and heavy. Focus on the feeling of heaviness, and suggest that your eyes will become so heavy and tired that you will close them and begin to enter a pleasant, relaxed state. After your eyes close, use any relaxation techniques you want to help you to achieve a deep, relaxed, hypnotic state. Here is a transcript of this procedure:

Select an object on which to concentrate. It can be anything simple, like a spot on the wall or ceiling, the flickering flame of a candle, or a ring on your finger. Focus on it. If your eyes should wander, just return your gaze to the focus object. Keep on staring at the object until your eyes become tired of it. Your eyes will probably begin to feel heavy . . . tired . . . so heavy that they feel like closing. You may feel drowsy . . . tired . . . feel like closing your eyes and entering a peaceful, relaxed state of mind. Feel yourself starting to relax. Then let your eyes close so you can begin to enter a pleasant, relaxed state.

Your breathing will start to slow down—a slow, deep, rhythmic breathing pattern. You're becoming more relaxed, more drowsy. You do not fall asleep; you just feel more relaxed—calm and relaxed. Your body is becoming loose, limp, and relaxed. Feel the relaxation spreading, all over, more and more.

A third hypnotic-induction procedure is the hand-levitation technique. Think of something that would make your hand light—so light that it could float. A common image is of a large helium balloon under the palm of your hand, making your hand light and buoyant. It could even be several helium balloons tied around your wrist, or one of your hands becoming a balloon pumped up with helium. Some other ideas could be imagining one of your hands as a piece of metal being drawn upward by the magnetic force of your head, which is an electromagnet, or your arm getting lifted by a series of ropes and pulleys that are being manipulated by you or someone else. Feel free to use your imagination in creating your own fantasies and suggestions. As the goal is hand levitation, use strategies that will result in such strong feelings of lightness that your hand and arm lift up.

Deepening Your Hypnotic State

Several methods can be used to deepen hypnosis. In the first transcript, we explored using pleasant imagery to deepen your hypnotic state. Suggestions of warmth and heaviness can also be used, or other methods, such as the stairway image and the counting technique. We will now describe several deepening techniques.

When using the stairway image, imagine yourself looking down a long stairway. Begin to descend, and with each step suggest to yourself that you are entering into a deeper state of hypnosis. Some people prefer elevators or escalators. Many people feel more in control if they have the freedom to choose how deep they will go. You can imagine that you are in control of the elevator, increasing or decreasing the depth of your hypnosis at the push of a button. If you are using the stairway image, you can imagine yourself going down as far as you wish. Some patients prefer to increase their hypnosis by imagining an elevator going up, although most people associate a deeper hypnotic state with going down. Use whatever you prefer. You can start by using the following transcript to practice deepening your hypnosis:

Now you can go into a deeper state of hypnosis. Imagine yourself walking down a long stairway. Picture each and every step you are taking. Each step you take helps you enter a deeper state of hypnosis. You can go as deep as you want by going down as many steps as you choose—down, deeper and deeper, every step taking you deeper. You are walking down, farther and farther, becoming more and more relaxed with each step.

If you would like to try using the counting technique as a deepening procedure, you should count from one to ten and suggest that, with each count, you will experience a deepening of the hypnosis. The following is a transcript for this procedure:

Now you are going to count from one to ten. During this count from one to ten you will be able to feel yourself going into a deeper state of hypnosis. One—the counting helps you to go deeper; two—each number brings you to a deeper level; three—letting yourself go as deep as you want; four—breathing slowly and deeply; five—with each count, each exhalation, you feel yourself becoming more relaxed; six—more and more relaxed; seven—deeper and deeper; eight—feeling yourself going even deeper; nine—deeper; ten—in a deep, state of relaxation, feeling so relaxed all over.

In using suggestions of heaviness for deepening hypnosis, suggest to yourself that various parts of your body feel heavy. You can use the following transcript:

Your arms are beginning to feel heavy. Your legs are beginning to feel heavy. Your entire body is feeling heavy. Your body feels so heavy that you feel yourself sinking into the chair, deeper and deeper. You feel yourself sinking into a deep, relaxed, hypnotic state.

Utilizing Hypnosis

The next stage is the utilization of hypnosis. After you have achieved a deep state of relaxation, you can give yourself therapeutic suggestions. Here are six general principles that can be used in the construction of most hypnotic suggestions:

1. Whenever possible, use positive wording in the construction of your suggestions. It is better to suggest, "I will feel pleasant sensations," rather than, "I won't feel pain." Be realistic. It is unrealistic to expect positive suggestions to perform magic or miracles. Therefore, suggestions such as "I will feel no pain" are to be avoided.

2. Use imagery as well as suggestions. Suggestions are more effective when you combine them with imagery. For example, in the case of relaxation, imagining a pleasant image such as a beach or mountain scene would help you become more relaxed than simply using suggestion alone. Using pain control as another example, if you wanted to create analgesia, you would use imagery as well as suggestions for producing numbness. You could imagine that you are receiving an injection of Novocain and suggest to yourself, "My hand is becoming numb; I'm feeling less and less sensation." You would continue to use the image and the suggestions until you obtained the desired result.

3. Make your suggestions flexible. Avoid "must's" and "should's". People often rebel when they are told, or tell themselves, what they "must" do. Therefore, avoid giving yourself rigid commands such as "I will never smoke another cigarette for the rest of my life." This type of suggestion is unrealistic, and it can create needless anxiety and depression should you fail to succeed perfectly and quickly. A more flexible suggestion would be, "I will become more and more in control over my desire to smoke as I learn to relax and cope with stress."

4. Allow time for change. Usually, changes in behavior and feelings occur over a period of time and in small incremental steps. Keep this in mind when you are formulating suggestions. Instead of expecting that you will stop smoking or eliminate pain overnight, give yourself suggestions that allow time to take place. For instance, a suggestion that allows for time would be, "As I continue to practice self-hypnosis, I will develop greater control over my feelings and experience more pleasant sensations."

5. Use repetition to increase the effectiveness of hypnotic suggestions. In addition to allowing time for change, repeat your suggestions again and again until they do have an effect. Practice self-hypnosis as often as you can. People often assume that hypnotic suggestions will continue to affect them indefinitely. Hypnotic suggestions can wear off. You need to reinforce your suggestions through repetition.

6. Avoid suggestions that imply failure or doubt. When constructing suggestions, avoid saying, "I will try to feel better," or "I'll try to give up cigarettes." "Try" implies failure. Give yourself the power. Suggest, "I will feel better because I will use my pain management techniques" or "I will quit smoking by using relaxation and self-hypnosis whenever I feel any craving."

There are several hypnotic interventions that are specifically used for pain control. We will describe three of these methods. They are hypnotic analgesia, dissociation, and suggestions for modifying sensations.

In using *hypnotic analgesia,* care should be taken not to mask pain that requires medical attention. This is usually not a problem because hypnotic analgesia typically wears off after a period of time and usually provides only temporary relief.

> *In using hypnotic analgesia, care should be taken not to mask pain that requires medical attention.*

In hypnotic analgesia, the patient experiences a dulling of pain. People who are most responsive to hypnosis may be capable of experiencing an absence of pain. Most patients are able to obtain some reduction in pain.

Suggestion and imagery can be used to produce hypnotic analgesia. While in the relaxed, hypnotic state, you can use the Novocain image described earlier. You can tell yourself to recall the feeling of Novocain or imagine an anesthetic lotion being applied to the painful area. Usually, the words "pain" or "painful" are to be avoided so that you focus on the numbness rather than the pain. The following is a transcript you can use to induce hypnotic analgesia:

The first step is to imagine that your fingers are becoming numb. You can imagine that you have just used a pleasant anesthetic cream on the fingers of one of your hands, and it is producing pleasant sensations. Notice whatever sensations are produced. You might be aware of a feeling of numbness in your fingertips or a tingling sensation. Just notice whatever change in sensation you experience.

Allow the sensations of numbness to spread to the rest of your hand. Your fingers are becoming more numb, and the numbness spreads to your hand. Your hand is becoming more numb. You are feeling less and less . . . becoming more and more numb. Now you can transfer the numbness to your stomach [use any body part that you particularly want to feel numb]. *You can now gently stroke your stomach and start to feel the numbness spreading from your fingertips to your stomach. Gently stroke the area and feel soothing sensations spreading from your fingertips to your stomach.*

Feel the numbness spreading and creating a very soothing, pleasant feeling. Whenever you want this feeling of numbness, just imagine this image: the feeling of numbness in your fingertips, then your hand becoming numb, and finally transferring the numbness to the area of your body that is causing you discomfort.

Dissociation, another hypnotic intervention, occurs when certain aspects of your experience are separated or "split off" from the rest of your consciousness. This occurs in everyday life when you become so absorbed in reading a novel or watching a movie that you become less aware of other events in the environment. In regard to pain, dissociation is what occurs when a wounded soldier is unaware of his pain until the battle is over, or when an athlete continues to play even though an injury has been sustained.

Most people are capable of experiencing dissociation to some degree. Combining imagery with dissociation can often facilitate this technique. You can imagine that you leave your body and go on a mental trip or go back in time to a pleasant memory. Your mental trip can be to your favorite place. This might be the pleasant image that you have already developed for relaxation. The following is a transcript of dissociation that can be used after you have achieved a state of deep hypnotic relaxation. This method works best if you tape-record your hypnotic induction, deepening techniques, and then the following transcript:

You are in a deep state of hypnosis and you can feel yourself drifting off, drifting off, and feeling detached—as if your mind were leaving your body. Imagine yourself leaving your body and floating . . . floating. You are looking down from above, observing your body with a sense of curiosity, feeling detached, as if you were watching someone else. You know it's you, but you feel detached, feeling more calm and in control.

Now imagine seeing yourself at the beach, [or whatever your image might be] *allowing yourself to drift off. You are drifting off into a deep, deep hypnotic state and feeling as if you were there now. Imagine being there now. See yourself at the beach, smelling the salt air, seeing the water, the sand, and the boats in the distance. You are now becoming less aware of your surroundings, less aware of yourself, less aware of your body. Just allow yourself to be totally absorbed by your image. Very relaxed, very peaceful.*

Another hypnotic intervention involves using suggestions to modify sensations. Instead of giving yourself suggestions to feel less pain, a more effective approach would be to give yourself suggestions to feel pleasant sensations. You can give yourself suggestions that create soothing feelings, such as coolness, warmth, or tingling. Use your personal preferences to select sensations that are soothing and pleasing to you. For one person, that would be warmth; for the next person, coolness. Remember, imagery increases the effectiveness of suggestions. If you want to create a feeling of warmth to soothe your pain, you might imagine the following image and give yourself the following suggestions after first achieving a deep state of hypnosis:

Imagine that you are sitting in front of a fireplace watching the flames. You enjoy watching the flames and listening to the crackling sound of the burning wood. You hold your hands out toward the fire, and you can feel the warmth. You feel the warmth of the fire against your body. It's so soothing, so comforting, so warm. You feel the warmth throughout your body . . . everywhere. You feel at peace. You feel good all over.

A modification of the above technique is to alter an unpleasant feeling, like a burning sensation, by gradually changing the intensity of the feeling. For example, if you experience your pain as a burning sensation, then suggestions of coolness could reduce the pain. Imagery helps here—a burning sensation could be given a color. If your pain had a color, what color would it be? One of our patients described his burning sensation as "red hot." His imagery incorporated the "burning red pain" as a starting point. While in a relaxed, hypnotic state, the following suggestions were given:

Imagine your pain as red hot. Now imagine the color is changing. The pain is cooling off with each exhalation, going from red to orange. With each exhalation you become more relaxed, and with each exhalation the color is changing gradually from red to orange. Now imagine it's changing from orange to yellow, gradually changing from orange to yellow, and becoming cooler. Now imagine it changing from yellow to a cool, neutral white. The yellow is fading, and as it fades you feel the soothing coolness.

Terminating Hypnosis

After you have given yourself suggestions for pain relief, you are ready to terminate your self-hypnosis session. Use one of the methods described earlier. Most people prefer to count from one to five and give themselves suggestions such as the following:

And now I will count from one to five, and by the time I reach the count of five, I will be fully alert and wide awake. I will continue to feel the [use whatever pleasant sensations you want to feel, such as numbness, warmth, or coolness].

One—slowly starting to return to the alert state; two—becoming more alert; three—starting to move my fingers and toes; four—becoming wide awake; five—opening my eyes, feeling wide awake and alert.

Feel free to experiment with the various techniques that we have described in this chapter. Be creative and modify any of our suggestions and transcripts so that they are consistent with your own preferences and style of language. They are only meant to be guidelines. Hypnosis is most effective when you are an active participant in the process. It's not magic, and it requires effort. You need to practice because it is a skill, but don't be intimidated. As mentioned earlier in the chapter, hypnosis is very similar to relaxation. If you can learn to relax, you can learn self-hypnosis.

This chapter has focused on methods for pain management. We know how difficult it can be for you to believe that you can control your pain, especially if that pain is not responding to medication. Ask for the medication that you need. If it doesn't work, be assertive and tell your physician. Perhaps the medication can be increased or changed. Maybe your physician can suggest other medical interventions such as electrical stimulation.

Even when pain cannot be eliminated, there is a good chance that, with the right combination of medication and pain control techniques, you will get at least some relief. Don't give up. Use the methods described in this chapter. Remember that hypnosis and other pain control techniques are not substitutes for medication. Use everything at your disposal.

6

Coping with Grief

Cindy came to counseling in order to prepare herself for her chemotherapy treatments. However, she was preoccupied with her anger toward her previous psychologist. He had insisted that she had to deal with her feelings about death, when what she wanted to focus on was what she needed to do to survive. Her previous psychologist said that she was resisting therapy and engaging in denial. He felt that she had to deal with her feelings now in order to be prepared for death.

When Cindy came to counseling with Dr. Bill Golden, she said, "I want you to help me do everything I need to do so that I can get through chemotherapy. I hope you won't make me focus on death like my previous psychologist. I want to focus on living. He said I would become depressed unless I deal with the issue of death right now. Do you agree?"

Bill explained, "There's a time to deal with grief, and obviously this isn't the appropriate time for you. You want to focus on what you need to do to increase your chances of survival. You're absolutely right in coming here to learn to deal with your anxieties about chemotherapy. At some later date you may need to deal with grief, but ultimately it's up to you to decide when that will take place." Bill then went on to teach coping techniques that helped control chemotherapy side effects and her anxieties about them.

Sometimes Denial Can Help

Cindy was engaging in what we would call *constructive denial*. Constructive denial is different from the defense mechanism of denial. Denial is harmful when it results in avoidance of feelings you need to face and actions you must take. For example, Cindy would have been engaging in the defense mechanism of denial if she avoided dealing with her anxieties about chemotherapy or avoided the treatment itself. We have heard patients actually say, "I'm not going to do any chemotherapy." On the other hand, constructive denial involves positive thinking and action that help you in coping with your illness. An example of constructive denial is the phrase that we've used previously: "Accept the diagnosis, defy the prognosis." In Cindy's case, her thinking and behavior were constructive in that they kept her focused on what she needed to do in order to maximize her chances of survival. The mistake made by her previous psychologist was that he was probably unaware of the constructive aspects of denial. He was trying to get Cindy to confront issues that she was not ready to acknowledge.

When is the appropriate time to deal with grief? The best time to acknowledge feelings is when you first begin to experience them. By acknowledging your feelings, you will be better able to cope with them. Denying your feelings will not make them go away. They could still bother you and might cause other symptoms such as anxiety, insomnia, headaches, and depression. Ultimately, the choice of when to deal with grief is up to you. No one can tell you when or how you should deal with life-and-death issues. Although there are typical patterns, people have diverse ways of dealing with grief. Keep in mind, however, that avoiding your feelings may also prevent you from exercising some of your options, thereby giving you less control of your life.

> *Denying your feelings will not make them go away.*

Edward described his feelings as "a heavy weight that was with me all the time until I came to terms with feelings about my death." By acknowledging his feelings, Edward was able to regain control: "I confronted my fear about dying. By facing my fear I started to come to terms with it. At first it was very unsettling, thinking about dying. However, over time I started to develop a new perspective. I realized everybody dies and that my time could be soon, so I'd better make the most of whatever time I have left. I started to make plans to do the things that I wanted to do. That's when I felt the weight lift. As I live my life more fully, I feel less afraid of dying. When it's my time, it's my time."

The Five Stages of Grief

According to Dr. Elisabeth Kubler-Ross, author of the book *On Death and Dying* (1969), there are five stages of grief: denial, anger, bargaining, depression, and acceptance. Patients with severe illness go through all, or most, of these five stages. Family members also go through a similar grief process. Stage one is denial, the stage in which you refuse to accept that you have a serious, life-threatening illness. Some patients avoid seeking treatment; others go shopping around for other doctors, hoping to hear that their previous diagnosis was incorrect. Why do people do that? Because denial can serve as a protective function. It can protect you from being overwhelmed by anxiety and despair when you are confronted by bad news. In the best-case scenario, denial allows you time to formulate a better way of coping with your diagnosis. In the worst-case scenario, denial becomes chronic, and the patient fails to come to terms with his or her illness.

Stage two is anger. You may feel resentment toward everyone around you, including your doctors. Displaced anger is when you cannot direct your feelings toward the actual source, and instead you "take it out" on everyone and everything around you. You may suddenly find that you become impatient with your spouse or other loved ones. It may seem as if no one is saying or doing the right thing. It's very common to resent people who are healthy. You may think, "Why did this happen to me? Why didn't it happen to him or her?" On the other hand, anger can mobilize you to take constructive action. Your family, friends, and doctors are not the enemy. Use your anger to fight your illness.

Stage three is bargaining. This is the stage in which many people turn to God, praying for a miracle or an extension of life. Religion and prayer can be very helpful in offering hope, and there is some evidence that prayer may have a healing effect. When David, the third author, was in the hospital prior to surgery for his brain tumor, he was visited by a rabbi and a nun. He found value in what both people had to offer. Although David was not deeply religious prior to his hospitalization, he found great comfort from both the rabbi and the nun. To this day, David thanks God for making each day beautiful, regardless of the weather. Even if it's raining, David is glad to be around for another day and continues to pray for more days to enjoy.

Stage four is depression and sadness. Sadness can be distinguished from depression in that depression is more severe and usually involves self-hatred, helplessness and hopelessness, or self-pity. Sadness, on the other hand, is the normal reaction to loss. It is part of the normal mourning process. Sadness or depression can occur in reaction to any loss. This can include the loss of the ability to function normally, the loss of a body part, the loss of a loved one, or anticipation of the loss of your own life. You can use the various coping strategies described in this book for coping with depression.

Stage five is acceptance. Acceptance involves finally coming to terms with the illness, and this can take considerable time and work. Acceptance is usually achieved as a result of expressing and resolving your feelings of anger and depression. It also involves making the most of whatever time you have left. The serenity prayer provides an excellent description of this stage: "God, give me the strength to change the things I can, the tolerance to accept what I cannot change, and the wisdom to know the difference."

Maintain Your Hopeful Attitude

Does acceptance mean that you have to give up hope? Absolutely not! You can be realistically hopeful, no matter what. How can you tell whether you are being realistic or engaging in "false" hope? No one can really say what false hope is, although some professionals are quick to offer opinions about it. For example, there are professionals in our field who have offered the opinion that Christopher Reeves, the star of *Superman,* may be offering false hope to spinal cord patients. Christopher Reeves is making a massive effort to seek a cure for spinal cord injuries, even though the skeptical professionals say we are not yet close to a cure. These professionals have criticized Christopher Reeves for building up the hopes of spinal cord patients, who will then be devastated when their hopes are not realized. The skeptics are saying that he is actually doing a disservice. We disagree! Even if someone has false hope, that's better than losing all hope. Once you lose all of your hope, you lose your will to live. So, better to have any kind of hope than none at all.

> *Once you lose all of your hope, you lose your will to live. So, better to have any kind of hope than none at all.*

There are many types of hope that you can have. With cancer, there is almost always realistic hope for a remission. In fact, almost every one of our patients has had one or several remissions. We believe that when you have hope and start to take control over your life and illness you have a greater chance of being a survivor. We have seen that patients without hope—those who have given up—die quickly. Hope is the springboard of the fighting spirit, and survivors fight.

It is realistic to hope for a better quality of life whether you are at the beginning stage of cancer, have been fighting for some time, or are at the final stage of your illness. Relief from both physical and emotional pain is possible. Sometimes pain cannot be completely eliminated, but it can be reduced to a manageable level. Most patients are able to experience relief from pain, if given adequate amounts of medication. As we mentioned in chapter 5, the research shows that physicians tend to underprescribe pain medication to cancer patients. If you are in pain, you need to be assertive and insist that you receive adequate amounts of medication. Depression can also be managed through antidepressant medication. Antidepressant medication can be used in combination with the depression-reducing methods described throughout this book.

Your Unique Experience of Grief

Many patients go through all five stages of grief. Others go through only a few of the stages. Knowing about these stages can be like having a road map. But don't feel you have to follow the map rigidly. For example, many patients experience only denial, sadness, and acceptance. In Edward's case, he experienced denial, then fear, and finally acceptance. Some patients return to earlier stages, such as feeling depressed again after a successful period of acceptance.

Miriam, after having accepted that she had a terminal illness, woke up one morning feeling depressed again. She couldn't understand why she had returned to this stage. She thought she had learned to cope with these feelings. She returned to counseling feeling very angry and depressed. "I can't understand why I'm going through this again. I thought I came to terms with my illness. Now I feel like I failed." Dr. Wayne Gersh explained, "It's something I see often in my patients who are struggling with serious illness. You don't necessarily go through those five stages of grief in sequence—it's an ongoing process. Sometimes depression follows a successful period of acceptance. Some of my patients have gone back to the denial phase and actually tell themselves they never had cancer. Some of these patients were successfully coping with anger and depression, and eventually did reach a level of acceptance. You haven't failed. It's par for the course. You can reach acceptance again."

Miriam felt some relief just knowing that what she was going through was not her fault nor so unusual. Wayne encouraged her to again use the coping tools for grief that we describe in this chapter.

As Edward's and Miriam's stories illustrate, not everyone goes through the five stages of grief in exactly the same manner. Nor is it written in stone that you must go through all of those stages before reaching acceptance. We will help you minimize depression and extreme anger, so you can move through them. Although there is a good chance that you will experience these emotions in coming to terms with your illness, you do not have to be stuck in those stages. We will help you to strive for acceptance and normal levels of grief so your quality of life can be improved.

Sadness and acceptance are not incompatible. As we said earlier, sadness is a normal part of experiencing grief and mourning. You can still accept that you have a serious illness and be sad about it. But your quality of life is likely to suffer if you start to feel depressed. You know you're depressed if you feel like giving up, lose all hope, or feel down all the time. Sadness, on the other hand, is less debilitating and does not have to interfere with the quality of your life. You can still experience joy and laughter, stay motivated, and continue to be optimistic and active, despite your sadness.

What determines whether you experience sadness or depression as part of grief? How you experience grief depends on how you view loss and how you respond to it. Many people who have become disfigured from surgery or have lost their hair to chemotherapy experience a loss of self-esteem and become depressed. But depression does not have to be your only option. Accepting yourself, regardless of how you may look physically, is the key to feeling sad as opposed to depressed. In chapter 7, we teach you how you can be more self-accepting.

> *How you experience grief depends on how you view loss and how you respond to it.*

A person can feel hopeless and helpless, or engage in self-pity in reaction to a diagnosis of cancer. Helplessness and hopelessness are the result of giving up. You are not helpless, even if you have cancer. As we described in chapter 2, you can develop a fighting spirit instead of thinking that you are helpless or that your situation is hopeless. Feeling sad will not prevent you from maintaining the fighting spirit. By fighting instead of giving up, you will fight depression as well.

It is perfectly normal that a person with cancer will feel sorry for himself or herself from time to time. However, excessive self-pity results in depression and anger. Self-pity can be identified by thoughts such as, "Poor me—why did this have to happen to me? Life stinks." The way to minimize self-pity is to focus on what is and what has been good in your life. Living life as fully as you can is another way to fight self-pity. This means getting out, continuing to be active, and even trying things that you have put off or never even considered. Instead of catastrophizing and thinking how awful it is that you have cancer, treat it as an opportunity. Use your grief about having cancer to grab as much life as you can, while you can.

Jeff felt hopeless and sorry for himself after finding out that he had metastatic cancer. Even though he was single, he rarely dated and had never had a significant relationship. Despite having an M.B.A., he had a low-level managerial position. He never applied himself—all his life he had coasted. After finding out that he had cancer, he began drinking excessively in an attempt to drown his sorrows. He was trying to come to terms with his grief over having cancer, but his method was self-defeating because drinking alcohol can increase depression and doesn't change anything.

When Jeff came to Dr. Bill Golden for counseling, he described what he was having as "a pity party."

"I've given up, and I know I'm feeling sorry for myself. I want to do something to improve my life, but I keep thinking, 'What's the use—I'm going to die anyway.' I was diagnosed five years ago, and I was told I wouldn't live for more than a year. So, I did everything wrong, because I thought doing otherwise would be pointless. The irony is that I'm still here. I guess I should stop feeling sorry for myself and do something constructive. That's why I called you."

Bill supported Jeff's view that by coming to counseling he had taken the first step in overcoming self-pity and helplessness. "It sounds like your drinking was an attempt to deal with your grief about having cancer. But it doesn't seem like it was an effective strategy."

Jeff replied, "I guess not. It did seem to make me more depressed and isolated. I would hang out in the bar drinking myself into a stupor. I'd see other people together and feel even more alone."

"There are better ways of dealing with grief. Most people go through what we call a stage of denial. Some people deny having cancer, while others deny or suppress their feelings. Your drinking was probably your attempt to suppress your feelings. It's okay to feel sad. You probably have to go through a period, or periods, of sadness. Acknowledge these feelings and try not to be terrified of them. If you allow yourself to experience the feelings, they will pass and you will be able to go on with your life. Even if you are sad, you can still set some goals. Goal setting is an excellent way of reducing depression. You will feel less sorry for yourself and less helpless as you pursue these goals. What do you think you would like to accomplish?" asked Bill.

"I know I need to stop drinking. I'd like to start dating because I'm lonely, and I'd like to look for a better job. I've been afraid to do these things, even before getting cancer. I guess now the attitude to take is that I have nothing to lose. I've always been afraid of rejection and failing. That's why I've never had a relationship and why I have the job I do," Jeff explained.

Bill agreed, "You have nothing to lose. You need to take risks. We can figure out a game plan where you will take small steps toward your goals. One way of reducing your anxiety about taking risks is to confront your fears one step at a time, starting with smaller, easier steps."

Bill taught Jeff the stress-management techniques, described in chapter 4, for reducing his anxiety. Jeff was able to stop drinking, begin socializing, and initiate a job search for a position that was more suited to his credentials. As soon as Jeff started to take action in pursuing his goals, his emotional outlook changed. Periods of self-pity were diminished. He rarely felt helpless because he could always focus on what he was doing to improve his life. At times, when he felt periods of hopelessness about the future, he reminded himself that he was doing more now to live life more fully than he ever had before. He allowed himself to experience all of his feelings, including sadness, and found that they did eventually pass. He was able to accept that he had cancer and that he might die from it someday, but at least now he was living life.

Sometimes making small changes in one's life is enough to overcome self-pity. In previous years, when Dr. David Robbins and his wife, Helene, went shopping together, she would pick his clothes for him. Her tastes were very conservative. When David first got his diagnosis of cancer, he went through a period of self-pity, regretting that he rarely made choices for himself. Finally, he decided that he was going to take control of his life and make decisions for himself—starting with selecting his own clothes. "Now that I have cancer, I don't know how much time I have left, and I don't know if I'm going to be here next year. Instead of feeling sorry for myself, I'm going to make the most of whatever time I have left and do it my way." He started by buying a fashionable coat of his own choice. This made him feel great, and he walked out of the store laughing. "I finally did it!"

Finally Letting Go

Hope for a cure or remission is usually absent when death is imminent. However, even when everyone has assumed that death is days or hours away, there are patients who have been able to make one final comeback. The question remains, if a patient is able to make one final comeback, is it worth it? Many family members have remarked to us that they wished their loved one did not have to suffer so much. For example, the Douglas family saw their son, Jonathan, struggling on his death bed. At the age of sixteen, Jonathan was hospitalized after having fought an aggressive cancer for many years. It was clear to both the family and the medical staff that Jonathan was at a final stage of his illness. The family was told that there was no further medical intervention, other than a morphine drip, to make him comfortable in his final days.

During the morphine drip procedure, nurses comforted him by talking to him and holding his hand. The family was convinced that they saw him die three times. They saw him close his eyes, appearing to pass into a sleep, and saw his breathing slow down to an imperceptible level. The monitoring devices were consistent with their perceptions; his breathing, heart rate, and blood pressure were depressed. Each time they thought he was gone he suddenly woke up, was alert, and spoke as if all was well. They heard him say, "I'm fine, I'm cured, I'm ready to go home." Then half an hour later, he slipped back into the nonresponsive state. This occurred three times. The family members all said they regretted having to witness Jonathan "dying three times." They wished it had been easier for him.

Some people argue that there is a time to let go of hope and life. Just as one's will to live can mobilize the body's resources for living, one can let go and welcome death. There is evidence that people are capable of willing their own death. We do not mean through suicide, but by giving up the struggle and accepting death in order to avoid further pain and suffering. We know of many people (including several of our relatives) who, after losing a spouse, said they lost their will to live and died shortly thereafter. One could argue that, because most of these individuals were elderly, there was a high probability that their death would shortly follow the death of their spouse. However, evidence of this phenomena occurring in younger people exists. During the Korean War, there were reports that some American prisoners of war, after being demoralized through brainwashing, just gave up and died. This occurred without any obvious physical cause. Psychologically induced death is also seen in cultures that are heavily steeped in voodoo and Santeria, such as in Haiti and Cuba.

If you can will your death psychologically, then why not just take matters into your own hands and kill yourself? Certainly, it's more efficient to overdose on your medication than it is to use your mind. Many people feel suicidal when they lose hope or feel chronic or intense pain. Some professionals and patient groups advocate for suicide as an appropriate option under these conditions. However, we believe there are better options. For example, most patients are able to experience relief from pain when given adequate amounts of pain medication. In addition, we have described pain control techniques that can be used in conjunction with medication.

We have seen that when patients exercise other options they later say that suicide would have been a mistake. Some of our patients were suicidal because they felt hopeless about ever feeling well again. With encouragement, they resisted their suicidal impulses and continued to fight their illness. Many of these patients later had remissions. Jim, for example, attempted suicide after a diagnosis of melanoma. A friend intervened and Jim was hospitalized. On the advice of his friend and the hospital staff, he went into counseling with Dr. Bill Golden. He began counseling feeling hopeless and scared. He explained that he attempted suicide because he was afraid of the pain and suffering he believed he was about to face. Jim asked Bill, "Isn't it rational to commit suicide under conditions like mine, where there is no hope?"

"You're assuming there is no hope. What is it that you feel hopeless about?" asked Bill.

"I'm never going to get better, and soon I'll be going through a lot of pain. I'll be a burden on my family," said Jim.

"Are you feeling any pain at this point?" asked Bill.

"No, but it's inevitable." answered Jim.

Bill explained to Jim that medication and psychological techniques could be used to control pain that he might experience in the future. "You probably can have a period of time where you can enjoy a decent quality of life. You would be losing out on that if you committed suicide now. I've seen many people in your situation who have enjoyed many good years, despite a diagnosis like yours. You are not at the last stage of cancer—you don't have any pain; you're able to function, and go to work, and even have fun. It's understandable that you're depressed. Who wouldn't be, after getting the news you just got? But I can help you with the depression, and I predict you won't be feeling suicidal once the depression lifts."

Bill helped Jim to recognize he wasn't hopeless and helpless. Jim realized there were a lot of things he could do and wanted to do while he was still able to function. He continued to work, socialize, date, and pursue his recreational pleasures. He even went back to school so that he could advance at his job. Clearly, in Jim's case suicide would have been a mistake. He was able to enjoy years of quality living before he became too sick to function. He continued medical treatments till the end, trying whatever he could to buy as much time as he could.

Although we recommend fighting your illness and using alternatives other than suicide, we do recognize that there may be a time when it is best to give up the struggle. Maybe the time to let go is when death is imminent—when you no longer have any strength and you are confined to bed. Is it better to go out peacefully, or fight to the last minute? We're not sure. Of course, this is a hard question for anyone to answer. Most of the time these decisions about whether or not to use heroic methods to maintain life are made at the last minute, which is not necessarily a good thing. The reason decisions about one's death are avoided is because of the extreme fear of death, especially in this culture. In eastern cultures, death is viewed as a natural part of life. People from those cultures are more accepting of death and are not afraid of it.

Religion and Spirituality

In our culture, many people are able to cope with their fears about death by using their belief in God and the hereafter. Mary found solace and comfort in the final stages of her illness through her belief in heaven. She was able to reduce her fears about dying by thinking about her mother and other loved ones whom she would be with when she died. Her belief in heaven helped her feel calmer and in control. She was able to accept death as part of the life process and used the following statements to reduce her fears: "There is no need to feel scared. Death is going to happen and when it does I'll be with God." Mary also used an image to help reduce her fear: She would imagine her mother in heaven smiling, with open arms, saying to her, "It'll be all right, I'm here for you."

For those of you who are not religious, there are other ways of coping with your fear of death. Ask yourself: What does death mean to you? Does the idea of death conjure up images of intense pain and suffering? Do you worry about how your loved ones will get through life without you? Some of your fears can be reduced through rational thinking and problem solving. In terms of pain and suffering, most of us really fear the process of dying, as opposed to death itself. From the scientific perspective, all pain and suffering end upon death. According to many scientists, once you die you feel nothing. In that case, you could view death as the end of suffering. The pain and suffering that you could experience as part of the process of dying can be controlled through pain medication.

Necessary Decisions

While it is probably not realistic for you to completely overcome your fear of death, you can prevent your fears from interfering with your decision making. Fear of death can interfere with major life decisions, such as preparing a will, estate planning, and deciding whether heroic means should be used to keep you alive at all costs. If you don't make decisions in advance about whether you want extraordinary means (such as life-support systems), then others will be forced to make those decisions for you. We have seen the extreme emotional pain that loved ones go through when trying to decide whether or not to permit medical staff to engage in heroic measures. You need to make your wishes known. Push past your fears, and take charge of your life—all aspects of your life—including your death.

Fears about how loved ones will go on after you die are quite legitimate, but solutions exist. Ironically, one of the advantages of a long-term illness is that it provides loved ones with a period of time during which they can learn to cope. In addition, you have the benefit of that time to resolve your own issues concerning death. In contrast, families who lose a loved one suddenly, such as in the case of a heart attack, are often in a state of shock and are ill-prepared. They have a harder time dealing with the loss because of their lack of preparation. You can be open and communicate with your family about your fears for them. You don't have to treat death as a taboo subject.

> Ironically, one of the advantages of a long-term illness is that it provides loved ones with a period of time during which they can learn to cope.

Talking about your fears and your family's fears can be very therapeutic. Communication about the possibility of death also allows for constructive problem solving. Very important issues, such as finances, college education for your children, estate planning, and your funeral can all be discussed. You need to make decisions that will probably be very important to you. You may not care much about your funeral arrangements, but most people, when they really start to think about it, have really strong feelings about where they will die, and with whom. Some people want the option of dying at home, in familiar surroundings. Rather than spending their last days in an impersonal hospital setting, they find comfort being with nurturing family members. This option does place a burden and responsibility on loved ones. Not only does it require an expenditure of time, but also a great deal of emotional support. Nevertheless, family members often reveal that they, too, found the experience rewarding and are thankful for having spent those last days together.

Hospice and Respite Care

Hospice care is another option. Certainly, hospice care is more pleasant than the hospital. Medical support is available and visitation is liberal. Hospice care can also help you to spend your last days at home with your family. The nurses, social workers, and other staff who offer their services through hospice care can facilitate and coordinate home care. They typically help the patient and the family utilize all the available community services. Family members are usually responsible for most of the actual care. Nurses educate the caregivers and monitor the patient.

We know of several families who utilized hospice care. In one case, hospice care enabled Joe to spend his last days visiting with his friends and his son, who had been away to college. Joe also had an opportunity to reconcile with his brother, whom he had not spoken to for several years.

The family recounts that instead of the hospice experience being gloomy, it was very positive. It had been years since the house had been filled with so many visitors, love, and laughter. It was a lot of work for the family, but there was also a lot of support from the nurse and the other hospice volunteers. The home care alternative also gave Joe the opportunity to spend one of his last days going for a drive in the country with his son, in his son's convertible.

Respite care is another resource available in many communities. Respite care allows family members to temporarily hospitalize their loved one. The temporary hospitalization enables family members to go on vacations or do other things that temporarily interfere with home care.

Although many patients find comfort in having family and friends around them in their final days, others want to die alone. Perhaps there are only certain people you want with you when death is imminent. You will probably want to make these decisions, rather than let others decide for you. Therefore, think about it and discuss your wishes with your family. Of course, thinking and talking about dying is very unpleasant and stressful. You will need to push yourself, and perhaps even your family, in order to get past the anxieties associated with this topic.

Unfinished Business

Fear about death can have a motivating effect. Use your fear to motivate yourself to enjoy life more. You can use the realization that you have limited time to encourage yourself to make the most of every day that you have left. Make every day count. Do all the things that you enjoy doing, including things that you have put off until tomorrow.

Take care of unfinished business. Most of us have unresolved issues with important people in our lives. There are "I love you's" that have never been said, apologies never made, phone calls never returned, "thank-you's" never written, and the list goes on. The reason why most of us have unfinished business is because of our fears. Another reason for unfinished business is benign neglect. We let other things get in the way of important priorities. Now is the time to take those risks and to take care of unfinished business.

Telling someone we love them involves risk because of our fear of rejection. At this point, what do you have to lose? Remember, you can feel good about yourself, being assertive and taking risks, no matter what the outcome. In all likelihood, you are not going to get rejected. We are talking about your expressing feelings to people who are an integral part of your life.

Jacob, for example, was never able to tell his son that he loved him. He never kissed him or gave him a hug. Jacob was inhibited by his belief that it was unmanly to show emotion. His son craved his affection, but was also unable to reach out. It wasn't until Jacob's diagnosis of cancer that he realized he was cheating himself and his son out of an important and loving experience. In counseling with Dr. Bill Golden, Jacob explored the reasons for his inhibition. He remembered how cold and aloof his father was. He thought that this was the way all men should respond. Nevertheless, he wanted to be closer to his son, and he realized he was running out of time.

Bill asked Jacob, "What are you afraid will happen if you take a risk, hug your son, and tell him you love him?"

"I don't know, maybe he'll pull away," replied Jacob.

"Do you have any idea how he feels about you?" inquired Bill.

"He tells my wife that he loves me a lot. She tells me he just isn't able to say it to me because he's afraid of the way I'll respond," explained Jacob.

"So you're both afraid of the same thing. You're both afraid to show how much you love each other. He's not going to reject you. It's just that you are both afraid. It's time to take the risk, Jacob. Let him know how you feel. You both deserve it," Bill advised.

At the next session, Jacob came in smiling, very pleased with himself that he had taken the risk. There were tears in his eyes as he described how he and his son hugged and told each other, "I love you." He said how hard it was for him to take that risk initially, but now that he had, he was able to say "I love you" every time he spoke to his son.

Jacob's case is an example of how you can make your life richer and more meaningful, despite limited time. Coming to terms with your mortality allows you to make the most of whatever time you have left. Facing your fears about dying will require great courage on your part. You don't have to deal with all of your fears at once. As we've tried to illustrate throughout this chapter, there are five stages of grief that you will probably go through. The process of acceptance takes time, so don't be concerned if you find that at first you are held back by denial or excessive anger. It's only natural that you will experience these roadblocks. They are part of the process. Be patient with your family, for they will also be going through these same stages. They may not be going through the process at exactly the same pace as you or be in the same stage as you. You will probably find it frustrating if you are ready to talk and deal with your mortality when your family is still in the stage of denial. Keep talking about your feelings. Don't let your family or friends stop you. Persist in trying to get them to deal with your feelings and your issues. Eventually, with patience, they will arrive at the same stage as you.

On the other hand, don't let family, friends, or your doctors push you into dealing with your death before you are ready to face it. Remember the case of Cindy. She was described at the beginning of this chapter as the woman who was angry at her previous psychologist because he insisted that she had to deal with her feelings about death. She was not ready to go through a grieving process. She was focused on what she had to do to maximize her chances of survival. Cindy had the right to decide when she was ready to proceed through the five stages of grief. So do you.

7

Loving Yourself

You may have heard the truism that says, Before you can love another person, you have to love yourself. The problem is that it's hard to feel any love when you are fixated on life-threatening issues. Because of your illness you may feel unlovable, that you don't deserve love, or that you are a burden to your family. You may assume that your loved ones find you unattractive or undesirable, or that they don't love you the way they did before you got cancer. These beliefs interfere with giving and receiving love. Very often they are based on false assumptions. When you are feeling vulnerable, it is very hard to check out your assumptions and communicate with family members to find out how they really feel. You can reduce that feeling of vulnerability by working on self-acceptance. When you accept yourself unconditionally and love yourself no matter what, you are better able to take risks. The focus of this chapter will be to show you how to develop greater self-acceptance and love yourself. Loving yourself will boost your positive, fighting spirit and enable you to reach out to others when the time is right.

Unconditional self-acceptance means that even if others reject or disapprove of you, you will still love and accept yourself. Having cancer makes it hard for some people to accept themselves. They buy into the notion that having a serious illness makes them

> *You don't become less desirable or less valuable as a human being because you have cancer.*

less desirable or less worthwhile. You can reject this self-defeating belief. You don't become less desirable or less valuable as a human being because you have cancer. Cancer did not transform your essence. You are still the same person you were before you got cancer. In order to achieve unconditional self-acceptance, you need to try to love yourself regardless of your health, regardless of whether other people love or accept you, regardless of whether or not you are successful, and regardless of whether or not you make mistakes. Love yourself in thought and action. It is just as easy to think positive thoughts as it is negative ones—don't condemn yourself. Fight those negative thoughts by using the techniques that we will be describing in this chapter. Treat yourself well. You deserve it. Act like you deserve to be treated well. Later in the chapter we will be discussing self-worth exercises. These exercises involve treating yourself with respect and dignity. Instead of beating up on yourself, be kind and considerate to yourself. Treat yourself like you are your own best friend. If you want to have love in your life, it's possible.

Anxiety and depression are the emotional obstacles that stand in the way of your getting the love that you want. As you know from previous chapters, negative thinking causes anxiety and depression. Low self-esteem involves a negative view of self and a tendency to " beat up" on oneself. Low self-esteem can be reflected by negative thoughts such as, "I'm unlovable now that I have cancer." "No one will ever want a woman with one breast." "I'm less of a man now that I have cancer." "I feel worthless now that I can't work." These negative thoughts cause depression. When you think less of yourself, you are likely to anticipate that others will criticize and reject you, thereby confirming your beliefs that you are worthless. Anticipating criticism or rejection will cause anxiety and avoidance. You are less likely to take the risks of showing affection, initiating sex with your partner, or sharing intimate feelings. We will show you how to overcome your obstacles.

Cognitive Therapy

Cognitive therapy is an effective approach for modifying negative thinking and depression. In chapter 3, we focused on depression stemming from pessimism and self-pity. In this chapter, the focus is on depression and anxiety resulting from low self-esteem. We will show you how to use cognitive therapy and other more active behavioral strategies for overcoming low self-esteem.

When using cognitive therapy, you identify your negative thoughts and you replace them with more positive, coping thoughts. Previously, we have described how to use a very simple technique called the two-column method. This exercise entails taking a piece of paper and dividing the page in half. You then record your negative thoughts on the left side, and substitute coping statements on the right side.

It may seem difficult for you to identify your negative thoughts at first. However, they might be right in front of you without your being aware of them. One of the easiest ways to uncover your negative thinking is to pay attention to your internal dialogue—your stream of consciousness. You will find that you are probably telling yourself negative things such as, "No one will ever want me—I'm unlovable." It often helps to write down these negative thoughts when you become aware of them.

Another way to get in touch with your negative thoughts is to think back to the situation that triggered your depression or anxiety. While imagining that situation, some of the negative thoughts about it will come to the surface. Write down these negative thoughts in the left-hand column.

> Be your own best friend.

The next step is to reevaluate these negative thoughts. Try to think of a more constructive way to think about that situation. Be your own best friend. If a friend was putting himself or herself down, what would you say to him or her? Would you agree with the put-down? Would you say, "Yes, you are worthless and unlovable?" Of course not! You would say, "Having cancer doesn't make you worthless and unlovable! You're still a good person." For every negative thought, write down a positive statement that you can use to counteract the negative thought. Not only should you write them down, but repeat them to yourself throughout the day. If you need a reminder, record them on an index card and review them periodically. The most important time to utilize your coping statements is when the negative thoughts pop into your mind. That is the time to fight and dispute them. Don't get discouraged if the negative thoughts keep returning. They probably will. Be prepared! Every time they return, remember to use your coping statements. They will work as long as you keep at it.

Iris: Using the Two-Column Method

Iris came to counseling feeling worthless. She gave up on love after her fiancé, Bob, ended their engagement when he found out that she had Hodgkin's disease. She became depressed and believed that she was stigmatized, worthless, and unlovable. Her medical treatments were successful, and her oncologist told her that she was cured. Nevertheless, she still felt inadequate. She was very depressed and felt hopeless about ever having love in her life again. The focus of her counseling was to help her to value herself despite having been rejected by her fiancé. With a little work, she began to realize that she did not have to accept this rejection as a judgment about her self-worth. She began to see that despite the illness and rejection, she was a valuable, desirable person who would be attractive to many other men.

Iris used cognitive therapy and the two-column method to help change her thinking. She was able to reject her negative thinking by developing coping statements. These coping statements were realistic, rational, and objective. They were not merely platitudes that would cause her to think positively just for the moment.

Situation: Bob Rejects Me

Negative Thoughts	Coping Statements
1. Having cancer is like having a stigma.	1. Having cancer is an illness, not a stigma.
2. I'm unlovable. No guy will ever want a woman with cancer.	2. I know that there are men who will not want me, but I also know that there are others who will find me attractive. I'm still a valuable, desirable person.
3. If Bob rejected me, I must be worthless. He was such a wonderful guy.	3. No matter who rejects me, I'm still worthwhile.

It would not have been helpful for her to merely tell herself that a man would accept her. Instead, she worked on accepting herself regardless of whether or not a man accepted her. Eventually, she was able to overcome her feelings of inadequacy and her fear of rejection, and she began dating again.

We will now use Iris's case as an illustrative example of the two-column method. Iris was able to identify her negative thoughts and arrive at coping statements that she used to reduce her feelings of worthlessness. The chart on the facing page is the one Iris used to improve her feelings of self-worth.

Now it's your turn. Use the following exercise to record your own negative thoughts about yourself, and construct positive, coping thoughts to counter them.

Two-Column Exercise

In the space provided, use the two-column method to list your own negative thoughts and compose alternative thoughts. Pick a situation in which you have difficulty accepting yourself, reaching out to other people, asking for what you want, or asserting your point of view.

Situation: _____	
Negative Thoughts	*Coping Statements*

Feelings of self-worth can also be changed by altering your behavior. We find that what we call "self-worth exercises" can be particularly effective as tools for promoting positive feelings. Self-worth exercises are action-oriented and entail treating yourself with worth, respect, and dignity. They can include giving yourself pleasure, being assertive, and taking control of your life.

Any pleasurable activity can be a self-worth exercise because it lets you know through action that you *deserve* to feel good. Be more self-nurturing. Don't wait for someone else to give you pleasure; give it to yourself. There are no universal exercises for self-worth. They are self-defined and self-determined. Only you know what will make you feel good. Just do it! Don't engage in self-denial. Don't postpone. You may not have the time later. Now is the time to act! Although you need to decide for yourself what is pleasurable, you can refer back to chapter 3 for a list of suggestions.

Assertiveness

Being assertive is another way of treating yourself with appreciation, respect, and dignity. Acts of assertiveness are affirming in nature because you are refusing to let anybody treat you with disrespect. In being assertive, you stand up for your rights without being hostile or putting the other person down. You are treating both you and the other person with respect and dignity. Assertiveness involves making requests, expressing positive and negative feelings, and confronting people who are being unfair to you. We will discuss how to be assertive later in this chapter.

By taking control of your life, you are saying that you are important enough to decide for yourself how you are going to live. Taking control of your life can involve very simple decisions that can make you feel better and make your life more pleasant. This can also involve major decisions that are concerned with life-and-death issues. For example, simple decisions can include deciding how and with whom you are going to spend your time, who your friends are going to be, and even what foods you might want to try. Some of the major decisions that you face may involve choosing between several treatments, choosing your doctors, and decisions about how you wish to be treated in the last stages of your life. Many of these decisions involve elements of assertiveness because in making decisions, you decide as opposed to letting others decide for you.

Monica: Problem Solving

Monica was faced with making the decision between a lumpectomy and a mastectomy. She was torn between her concerns about the possibility of metastatic cancer and losing her breast. The first surgeon she saw was vehement in his advice to her that she should undergo a mastectomy. His position was that a lumpectomy increases the risk of metastatic cancer. She went for a second opinion from a surgeon who supported her right to choose a lumpectomy as an alternative. His position was that although there are risks, lumpectomies can be effective without metastatic recurrence in cases like hers. She was torn between these two options, and this was further aggravated by her family members who were putting pressure on her to get a mastectomy.

Monica's psychologist, Dr. Bill Golden, supported her right to choose for herself and helped her to make a rational decision. She was shown how to use the problem-solving technique that we first described in chapter 1. First, the problem was identified. Monica defined the problem as, "What should I do about the lump in my breast?" Through brainstorming, they listed all of the various alternatives. These alternatives were identified as mastectomy, lumpectomy, chemotherapy, or radiation therapy. The next step was to look at the advantages and disadvantages of each choice. This involved doing research. Monica found that having chemotherapy or radiation without surgery were not acceptable choices for her because of the high recurrence rates. She chose the lumpectomy combined with chemotherapy because there were enough data supporting the efficacy of that procedure, given her physical condition. She had no lymph node involvement, and the tumor was confined to a small area. The combination of the medical data and her desire to keep her breast outweighed the advantage of a mastectomy, which can lead to a reduced risk of recurrence. Monica felt empowered by her realization that she could take control of her life. In Monica's case, a positive outcome resulted, as she is still alive today. However, regardless of the outcome, the right choice for Monica was to make the choice her own and to be assertive. Nevertheless, Monica's decision is not necessarily the right decision for everyone. Each case needs to be evaluated in terms of medical advice, research relevant to your particular case, and your personal feelings.

Monica realized that in order for her to take charge of her life, she needed to take risks. Not only was she taking a risk with her life, she was risking the disapproval of family members and a reputable physician. Assertiveness, decision making, and taking charge of your life involve risk taking. Risk taking requires self-acceptance. Taking risks implies that you may fail, that you may make a mistake, or that people may disapprove of you or reject you for your choices. You need to be able to accept yourself, regardless of the outcome. You do not become less worthwhile if you make a mistake, fail, or get rejected. You are the same person, and you have the right to make decisions for yourself regardless of what other people think. The consequence of letting other people decide for you and judge you is to feel less worthwhile. You are at the mercy of others if you let your feelings of self-worth be determined by other people. Feelings of worth can be increased by taking risks, taking charge of your life, and being assertive. We will now discuss how you can be more assertive.

> *In being assertive, you express feelings without attacking other people or putting them down.*

A distinction could be made between assertive, nonassertive, and aggressive behavior. In being assertive, you express feelings without attacking other people or putting them down. You stand up for your rights while respecting the rights of others. You're direct and appropriately honest, you take responsibility for your feelings, and you choose for yourself. You use "I" statements in expressing your feelings. For example, "I feel annoyed when you try to tell me what to do." You also make suggestions rather than tell people what to do. For example, "I would prefer to make the decision myself."

Nonassertive or passive communication is indirect and emotionally dishonest. You don't tell the person how you really feel. If you do express yourself, it is often in an indirect manner, without taking responsibility for what you really want. An example of nonassertiveness would be the following: You really want to go out for dinner and eat pizza. You ask your spouse what he or she feels like eating, without saying what you would like to eat. In other words, asking without requesting. If you request, you state your position; if you ask, you do not say what you really want. In being nonassertive, one avoids taking responsibility for one's feelings and allows others to choose instead. Nonassertive behavior is self-denying and inhibited, and usually does not get you what you want.

Aggressiveness is direct and honest communication, but in a hostile manner. You express feelings without editing. You attack the other person, putting him or her down, perhaps engaging in name calling. Not only do you make choices for yourself, you make choices for others without respecting their feelings. You may achieve your goal by being aggressive, but at others' expense.

Here are several guidelines for acting assertively:

1. When expressing your feelings, use "I" statements.

2. Don't attack the other person or make global evaluations. Comment on their behavior. For example, "I feel annoyed when you tell me what to do" instead of "You're always telling me what to do."

3. Make suggestions, and tell the person what you would like them to do instead of making demands and telling them what to do. For example, "I would appreciate your coming with me to my doctor."

4. Express your feelings calmly. Avoid yelling or name calling.

5. When refusing another person's request, be clear and decisive. You can give an explanation, but don't be overly apologetic. For example, Joy was assertive with her husband who continued to expect her to do the same amount of cooking and cleaning despite her great fatigue from her chemotherapy and postsurgical discomfort. She said, "I wish I could do what I used to, but I just can't. I don't have the energy that I used to."

6. You have the right to refuse help. It's okay to set limits with well-meaning family and friends. For example, "I appreciate your wanting to help me, but I feel quite capable of doing it on my own."

7. If someone asks you to do something that you believe is unreasonable, request an explanation. For example, "Why do you expect me to just get over it and be happy all the time? I think it's reasonable for me to be sad sometimes."

8. Strive for assertive body language and tone. Maintain good eye contact. Avoid whispering or being overly loud.

9. As you learn to become more assertive, you are likely to experience discomfort. That is because as you take risks, you confront your fears. Think of it as growing pains. It's going to take time and practice before you feel comfortable being assertive.

10. Use imagery to mentally prepare yourself for difficult situations. Mentally rehearse what you would like to say.

11. Remember, be kind to yourself. In the process of being assertive, you will make mistakes. Don't get angry at yourself if you should behave nonassertively or aggressively. Instead, figure out what you did wrong, and think about how you could be more assertive next time.

Keep in mind, even if you follow all of these guidelines, there's no guarantee that you will get what you want. The other person has just as much right to refuse your requests. If you find it difficult, remember that there are many reasons to be assertive: You are more likely to get what you want by being assertive than by being passive. Feelings of self-respect and respect from others will result from being assertive, regardless of whether you get what you want. We teach other people not to respect us and to take advantage of us when we are unassertive. By being assertive and telling other people how we feel, we are giving them the benefit of the doubt and allowing the possibility of an improved relationship. The relationship can become more authentic and satisfying to both parties.

There may be reasons why you have trouble being assertive. Fear of disapproval and rejection are common themes. Most of us wish to be approved of and loved by others. However, needing love and approval in order to feel worthwhile will lead to anxiety and unassertiveness. You need to confront your fears and take risks. Accept yourself whether others approve or not. Believe that what you feel is right because you feel it and because you have the right to tell others how you feel.

Another common fear is the fear of being imperfect, failing, or looking foolish. We can tell you right now that you will make mistakes in the process of being assertive. It's impossible to be perfect when you are first learning a new skill. Understand that assertiveness takes time and it involves practice. It's better to risk making mistakes and looking foolish than to be passive. Passivity will not get you what you want. Taking a risk and looking foolish, on the other hand, will give you the learning experiences you need in order to improve. You may think you look foolish, but compared to what you were doing before, you will probably simply look more assertive to other people. So take the risk and start the learning process. You will get better with time and practice.

Feelings of guilt may be another reason you may have difficulty being assertive. The "guilt trip" occurs when you think that you're bad and that you are doing something wrong by being assertive. While it is true that someone might feel hurt as a result of your assertiveness, you have the right to act in your best interests as long as your intent is not to purposely hurt the other person. For additional help in learning to be assertive, consult Dr. Herbert Fensterheim and Jean Baer's book, *Don't Say Yes When You Want to Say No* (1975).

Anna had trouble being assertive with her oncologist because she felt very intimidated by the doctor. The doctor was evasive whenever Anna tried to get information about her condition and treatment. Anna was afraid that the doctor wouldn't like her and would abandon her if she persisted in asking questions. In addition, she was doubting her right to obtain this information and thought she might be a "pain in the ass."

Anna was already in treatment with Dr. Bill Golden for learning to cope with chemotherapy side effects. During one of her therapy sessions, Anna mentioned her difficulty with the oncologist and asked for help in coping with her fear about being assertive. With Bill's help, Anna was able to identify the thoughts and feelings that were preventing her from being assertive. She was experiencing a combination of anxiety and guilt. The negative thoughts associated with her anxiety were, "The doctor won't like me. The doctor will abandon me. I won't get treated properly, and I'll die." The negative thoughts associated with her guilt were, "The doctor is right, I'm badgering him. I'm being a pain in the ass."

Bill introduced the two-column method to Anna. The two of them collaborated in coming up with coping statements that helped Anna reduce her anxiety and guilt enough to be assertive with her oncologist. The two-column method containing Anna's negative thoughts and coping statements can be found on the following page.

Imagery and role-playing were used to give Anna additional help in being assertive with her doctor. Anna used imagery to mentally rehearse what she would say to the oncologist. She also rehearsed her coping statements, imagining what she would say to herself to help her be more assertive. In addition, she and Bill role-played her being assertive with her oncologist. Anna found role-playing very helpful in preparing her for her discussion with the oncologist. At first, the oncologist was again evasive, but Anna

Situation: I Am Assertive with My Doctor

Negative Thoughts	Coping Statements
1. The doctor won't like me.	1. The doctor doesn't have to like me. I have the right to ask him questions.
2. The doctor will reject me, I won't get treated properly, and I'll die.	2. My doctor is one of the best in his field, but he is not the only one. It's unlikely that he would abandon me because that would be unprofessional conduct.
3. The doctor is right— I'm badgering him. I'm being a pain in the ass.	3. Patients have the right to ask questions about their condition and treatment whether the doctor likes it or not.

persisted. Finally, the oncologist answered her questions and seemed to be more responsive in future discussions.

In Anna's case, Bill role-played the oncologist. What you can do is develop your own coping statements using the two-column method. For practice with being assertive, you can request help from a friend or family member, asking them to role-play with you. This, in itself, is practice in being assertive because you are making a request. Hopefully, as a result of your assertiveness, your friend or family member will help you. Keep in mind that assertiveness doesn't guarantee that you will get what you request. Other people have a right to be assertive and refuse.

Use the exercise below to map out specific actions you will take to think more positively and act more assertively.

Your Assertiveness Plan

Pick a situation in which you are having trouble reaching out to others, asserting your rights, or accepting yourself in relation to others. Use the two-column method as a springboard to an assertiveness plan. In the first two columns of the chart on the following page, proceed as usual by writing down your negative and alternative coping thoughts. Then write down what you will say, what you will do, and with whom you might role-play the scene.

Situation: _____				
Negative Thoughts	Coping Thoughts	What I Will Say	What I Will Do	Role-Play With

Teri: Using the Assertiveness Plan

Teri was a single, thirty-one-year-old woman who was feeling depressed and unlovable after her mastectomy and chemotherapy. Her hair, once lush and luxurious, was still very thin and lifeless. She covered it with a scarf at all times, even when she was alone. She felt ugly and worthless after reconstructive surgery that left her with a new breast that was higher, harder, and rounder than her other breast. She felt that she no longer looked natural and that any man who saw her naked would be "grossed out" by her appearance.

She was scheduled to return to work in two weeks and dreaded walking into the office wearing a scarf. She didn't want to buy a wig because she felt it would look artificial and everyone would know she had cancer. She needed to consider which specific thoughts and actions would help her through her re-entry period at work. With the help of her psychologist, Dr. Bill Golden, she construct an assertiveness plan, which follows:

Situation: Walking into Office Wearing a Wig

Negative Thoughts	Coping Thoughts	What I Will Say	What I Will Do	Role-Play With
They'll see I look phony and know I have cancer.	*No mind reading—I can't predict what others will think.*	*"Hi. Gosh I'm glad to be back! Tell me everything I've missed."*	*Get a really good wig that looks like my old hairstyle.*	*Grace.*
They'll shun me.	*Give people a chance.*	*Ask Marsha and Shirl out to lunch.*	*March right into my cubicle, smiling and nodding to everyone.*	

I'm worthless.	I'm the same worthwhile person I always was.	"It's been difficult, but the worst is behind me. I want to focus on the future."	Change the subject if necessary.	

Teri spent $400 on a wig that closely matched her precancer hair color and texture. She had it trimmed and restyled to match her old hairstyle. She wore it around her apartment until she could stop touching and adjusting it, and no longer glanced into every mirror and reflective surface to see how it looked. Her sister Grace went out to lunch and shopped with her so that Teri could get used to appearing in public with the wig. While they were out, Teri practiced the things she planned to say when she went back to work.

On the morning of her return to work, Teri dressed carefully and wrote her coping thoughts and statements on some index cards. She slipped them into her purse and drove to work. She was very nervous parking her car and walking toward the building, but as soon as she opened the door she felt better. Her preparation for being assertive made it seem like she was in a well-rehearsed play, where she knew what she would say and do next.

After her successful return to work, Teri told her psychologist, Bill, "Although I feel more comfortable with my wig, I could never let a man see my breasts. What if I met someone I really cared for, and he rejected me?"

He suggested that she read Betty Rollin's book, First You Cry (1993). Teri learned that many women with breast cancer share her concerns. With Bill's encouragement, she worked on her fears of rejection and she used her assertiveness planning skills to gradually start dating again, taking it very slowly.

Teri worked on her self-deprecating thoughts. She made a plan for what to say and do so that she could just leave her bra on during sex. In fact, she kept her bra on through two relationships. Although the men were obviously curious, they never demanded an explanation, never mentioned the bra, and remained interested in her.

Eventually, Teri met a man she really liked and trusted. She took the risk of talking about her mastectomy and fears of rejection. Finally, in an intimate setting with candlelight, music, and incense, she was able to remove her bra and be seen. It was worth the risk.

The main focus of this chapter has been to help you to love and accept yourself. By loving yourself, you will be able to love others. You will also be able to take the risks that increase the feelings of empowerment and competence that will help you to fight your illness. The methods and techniques that we have offered you will be valuable tools for reaching out. In the next chapter we will be helping you to get the love and support that is so valuable in coping with stressful situations and illness.

Reaching Out

Although it may be difficult to think about feelings of love when confronted by a serious illness, they can be a great source of pleasure and support. Throughout this book we have been emphasizing how important it is to enjoy life to the fullest. Life doesn't stop when you have cancer. Nor does love have to stop when you have cancer. Receiving love, care, and support are very important in coping with cancer. We have seen that receiving love and support, whether coming from a marital partner, family members, or friends, helps patients adjust to their illness. John found that having his wife's love and support was reassuring and inspirational. He could depend on her to take care of details concerning his illness and everyday life, freeing him from some of his worries. Her helpfulness allowed him to focus more of his time and attention on recovery. Her love, as well as their children's, gave him meaning and purpose for living and fighting his illness. Therefore, reaching out to others and allowing others to reach out to you will not only improve your quality of life, but will also help you to cope with your illness.

The focus of this chapter will be on the emotional support that you can receive from family and friends. In the preceding chapter we mentioned how low self-esteem could interfere with giving and receiving love. In this chapter, we will be focusing on the various emotional inhibitions that interfere with communication and intimacy. We will show you how to break down the barriers that may have developed between you and the people in your life.

The Web of Silence

Serious illness often results in a web of silence. Your family, your friends, and even you may find it very difficult to communicate. The people around you may seem like a bunch of phonies. They may be assuming a mask of cheerfulness and avoiding discussion of your illness. Many people shy away because your illness reminds them of their own mortality. They're also afraid they will say the wrong thing—that they will offend you or cause you to feel upset.

Phyllis came to counseling feeling extremely isolated. Most of the people in her life were unable or unwilling to let her discuss how she felt about her illness. Every time she tried to talk with her husband about her worries and sadness he would say, "Everything is going to be all right. Stop worrying. Don't be so negative and you'll be okay." Whenever she would see her best friend, Melanie, the conversation was about everything but her illness. Melanie would ask, "How's your job? Are you going on vacation? How are the kids? How's your husband's diet?" Melanie never asked, "How are you?" When Phyllis went back to work as a school teacher, only one teacher was willing to talk with her about her illness, despite the fact that most people in the school knew. Her principal could not even look her in the eye. When Phyllis came for counseling, Dr. Wayne Gersh encouraged her to express her feelings. She remarked that she felt so relieved and said, "Thank you for letting me be depressed. This is the first time anyone has allowed me to talk about my feelings." After Phyllis talked to Wayne about her feelings, she then expressed interest in learning how to cope. People are generally more receptive to problem solving and positive thinking after they have had the opportunity to vent their feelings.

Wayne helped Phyllis deal with her feelings of isolation. He recommended that she start with her husband by teaching him how to be a better listener. "You can tell your husband, 'Just listen. I don't need solutions right now, I need you to listen.' Your husband will probably resist because he believes he is doing the right thing and believes that he is listening."

Phyllis was able to get her husband to listen. At first, he did get defensive. But eventually he understood that his giving advice was not the support his wife wanted.

There is a time for advice and a time to just be a supportive listener. Who decides when is the right time for listening or advice giving? You do! If you want advice, you can ask for it. If you want others to listen, you can ask for that as well. Don't assume that they know what to give you. They will respond in the way that is typical of them. You need to assume the responsibility of teaching them what kind of communication would be most beneficial to you at a given time. You could try the same approach with friends and associates. Of course, it can be more difficult to allow yourself to be vulnerable with them. They could get defensive: "I'm trying to help you"; "I'm not your therapist"; "Don't you have a husband for this?" are some of the statements you may hear. They may withdraw from you. They may even gossip about you and tell all your mutual friends, "That cancer has really changed her. She's so aggressive. It's not nice being around her."

As we said in the preceding chapter, assertiveness involves risk taking. You might get rejected or face disapproval. That does not make you a bad person. You have a right to express your feelings and ask for what you want. You will find out who your real friends are. Don't be shocked if most of the significant people in your life have trouble talking with you about your illness. As Phyllis discovered, most of the people in her life disappointed her. This is not that unusual. Most people have limitations. Be careful that you don't reject everyone. If you reject everyone who disappoints you, you will end up alone. In deciding who to accept with their limitations, ask yourself, "Does the good outweigh the bad?" Assuming all friends and loved ones have limitations, it is up to you to decide what form of limitations you wish to accept.

One reason why family, friends, and associates might be acting as if everything were okay is that they are afraid that you will become upset or seriously depressed if negative feelings are acknowledged. To most people, you are seen as the person that must be kept happy at all costs. Another possible reason is the mistaken belief that negative feelings are dangerous to your health. They may have read or heard that depression reduces one's ability to fight an illness. They may know that being positive can improve one's chances of survival. In fact, they are both right and wrong.

As we have said throughout this book, maintaining a positive outlook will help you fight depression, anxiety, and cancer. Nevertheless, denying negative feelings is neither helpful nor therapeutic. Expressing your feelings is a cornerstone in your battle against cancer. This may sound like a contradiction, but it's not. Positive thinking and expressing negative feelings are both therapeutic strategies that have their time and place. You need to acknowledge what's bothering you before you can do something to change. Identifying what you're thinking and feeling is the first step in cognitive therapy, prior to reevaluating and changing your outlook. To entertain only positive thoughts is like walking down a street and not knowing where you are going.

The Importance of Catharsis

Another reason for acknowledging and expressing your negative feelings is to achieve a catharsis, or emotional release. There can be therapeutic value to venting your feelings instead of bottling them up. Reaching out to family and friends can provide you with an opportunity for a cathartic experience.

When Dr. David Robbins was first diagnosed with a brain tumor, he and his wife spent many hours discussing their fears. He was afraid of dying and leaving his wife. He was afraid that his daughters would grow up without him. At first his wife, Helene, offered reassurance, "You'll be all right, you're not going to die. You won't leave us." David knew that Helene was trying to get him to think positively and do all the right things to help himself, which David was already doing. It wasn't what David needed at that moment. So he said, "I just need you to listen. There's so much on my mind that I just want to get out—please listen." Helene was very responsive and let David talk about his fears. In reflecting on this experience, David has said, "I really got a lot out that was on my mind. It was a real relief to talk about it."

However, you may feel that you don't want to burden your family and friends with your feelings. This is a common concern, based on the belief that family and friends are already over-whelmed by your medical condition. Many people are unable to express their feelings out of guilt. They incorrectly think it would be too self-indulgent or selfish. You may also be incorrect in your thinking. Maybe you are jumping to conclusions. Family members may welcome the opportunity for everyone to speak freely. They may be avoiding discussing any feelings because they may be afraid that this will upset you. By your initiating communication, you are giving them permission to acknowledge feelings.

Carol came to see David to discuss feelings that she felt unable to express to her family. She had advanced lung cancer and felt that there was little time left. At the end of the first session, she thanked David for listening. She said, however, that she did not know when she could come back because she did not want to be a burden to her family.

David raised the question, "How do you know that it would be a burden to them?"

Carol said, "I'm just assuming it. I've been so much trouble to them already."

David then asked, "Is that also the reason why you don't talk to them about your feelings?"

"Absolutely!" she said. "Who wants to hear about my fears about dying? I don't want to burden you with them either."

David then pointed out that Carol was assuming that she would be a burden to both him and her family. He pointed out that she was not allowing herself to get the help that she needed and had the right to obtain. "Carol, you are assuming that everyone will be burdened by your feelings. You are jumping to conclusions. For example, you're thinking I will be burdened. This is my job. I do it all day. I want you to express your feelings. I welcome them. And if you're making these false assumptions about me, then maybe you're doing the same thing with your family. How could we check out your assumptions to see if they're true or not?"

Carol said, "I guess I could ask them, but I'd feel so guilty."

"What would you be guilty of?" David asked.

"Burdening them," she said.

"You really seem to have a thing about burdening people. Where does that come from?"

Carol then told her story.

"My mom died when I was six or seven. My dad worked very hard and told me he couldn't take care of me. 'You're going to stay with Aunt Theresa and Uncle John.' Life with them was very hard. They had five kids of their own and they were burdened—and they let me know it. I was always doing things to help out while their other children were having fun. I had to earn my keep. That's the way my life was until I met my husband, Anthony. At that time I thought my life would change, but it didn't. Anthony, who is a doctor, left for the hospital very early in the morning and didn't come home until late at night. I got pregnant and my son was born. Raising him took all my time. When my son was two, I got pregnant again. This time I had a girl. My workload was doubled. I never asked for help; I just assumed I should take care of it all myself. I got the cancer when the kids were grown up and already working. This was the time that I thought would be mine, and now I have to deal with having cancer."

After listening very carefully to her story, David said to Carol, "No wonder you have trouble asking for help. As a child you were told you were a burden. You spent your whole life helping and doing for others. You never had the chance to take care of your own needs. Everyone has needs, and everyone has the right to ask for help. That's not being a burden. With your background, I could understand why you feel like you're always burdening others. But you do so much for others. Now it's your turn. Stop assuming Anthony is just like your aunt and uncle. Take a risk and ask for help. If Anthony doesn't respond in a positive way, it doesn't mean that you're wrong."

That week Carol spoke to her husband about his taking her for more counseling. She also expressed her fears about her illness to Anthony. On both counts he was responsive. Carol also talked about how she felt she was being a burden to him. Anthony told her that he wanted to do more for her and her opening up allowed him to be more responsive. Although Anthony never became the most supportive husband, Carol felt that she was better able to communicate with him.

When Not to Reach Out

Sometimes reaching out does not work. Sometimes, a family member or friend is unable or unwilling to be supportive. Harriet was in this position. Like Carol, Harriet came to David because she felt a desperate need to talk. She was being treated for a brain tumor and was undergoing chemotherapy. Harriet tried to talk to her alcoholic husband about helping her with issues surrounding her illness. He refused to be supportive in any way. He never visited her in the hospital when she was first diagnosed. He refused to drive her to her chemotherapy or radiation therapy. He even refused to hear anything about her illness.

Harriet was more depressed about her husband's reaction to her than she was about her cancer diagnosis. She blamed herself for his drinking and withdrawal from her. She felt that her cancer contributed to his drinking and that she shouldn't burden him.

After listening to her story, David agreed that she could not look to her husband for support, but she was not to blame for his excessive drinking and rejection of her. These were his problems independent of her illness and were symptoms of alcoholism. She needed to look at other alternatives for support and nurturance. David recommended that she reach out to her daughters, who were already supportive. He felt that she could spend more quality time with them, rather than wasting time trying to get her husband to change. He also recommended the American Cancer Society, Al-Anon (a support group for family members of alcoholics), and her church.

After attending several support group meetings, she came back to counseling and said to David, "Wow, I never realized there were people out there who cared. Actual strangers were willing to listen, give advice, and most important, be my friend. I also have my daughters to help me through this. They're more wonderful than I anticipated."

As illustrated by Carol's and Harriet's cases, you need not ever feel like you're a burden. Even if someone else feels that your illness is a burden to them, that's his or her problem. The problem posed by an unresponsive husband, wife, lover, or friend is real. But, you don't have to blame yourself. You have a right to reach out, to seek help and emotional support. The solution is to look for that support from receptive, caring people, whoever they may be. If they are not in your home or your present social network, then reach out to support groups or professionals trained in counseling cancer patients.

Gender Differences

Although you have a right to seek emotional support from significant others, keep in mind that there are gender differences between men and women in communication styles. It has been observed for years by both psychologists and marital counselors that men and women differ in the ways they communicate. Men tend to focus on being solution-oriented in their approach, while women are more satisfied by expressing their feelings. This gender difference is often the source of conflict for couples. June, for example, was feeling quite frustrated because when she expressed her fears about a possible recurrence, her husband, Donald, kept reminding her of all the treatment alternatives. He wasn't purposely trying to frustrate her—he was communicating in a way that is typical for most men. He thought she was obsessing and whining instead of being rational, like him. They ended up arguing instead of communicating. They were too focused on who had the correct approach, problem solving or expression of feelings. He thought she was a whiner; she thought he was cold and uncaring.

They remained locked in this power struggle until they came to counseling. Dr. Bill Golden explained to them that their communication pattern was almost universal. Men tend to look for solutions and prefer problem solving as a communication style, whereas women derive therapeutic benefit from having a sympathetic listener. The key is to work as a team and be respectful of each other's communication style. There is a time for expressing feelings and a time for problem solving.

Donald objected to Bill's advice at first. "That sounds so unproductive and inefficient. I don't see how focusing on a recurrence is going to help her to feel better. That sounds very negative to me. You may be right that women think like this, but if they do they should be more like men."

Bill responded, "First of all, it's not always the case that women prefer to express feelings and men problem solve. There are many cases where the opposite is true. Nevertheless, you are assuming there is a right and a wrong way of dealing with feelings. Whatever works for a given individual is the right way. What is your goal, anyway?"

"To help my wife, of course," said Donald.

Bill went on to say, "Then it's up to June to decide what would be most helpful in this case. If you were the one with the problem, then you could decide what would be most helpful."

Donald was able to respect June's desire to express her feelings without his offering solutions. He worked hard at being a good listener. June became more patient with her husband when he started to give advice because she now knew that this was his communication style. She no longer felt that he was trying to control her.

Being Assertive with Overprotective Caregivers

Good intentions can result in good or bad outcomes. In the beginning of the chapter, we discussed the case of John, who found it very helpful to be able to depend on his wife's willingness to take care of details concerning his illness. Her helpfulness allowed him to focus more of his time and attention on feeling well again. On the other hand, too much help can make someone feel helpless. Family, friends, or associates can hurt you in spite of their good intentions if they treat you like a helpless cripple. Their intentions are to help or protect you. They think you need to conserve your energy in order to fight your illness. The reason they are doing things for you that you could do yourself is that they are trying to help you, or help you "save face."

Shirley kept trying to protect Harry from failing at activities that, prior to cancer, he was able to perform. Although Harry was still capable of most of these activities, Shirley was afraid that he would fail or that he might be embarrassed because he might not be as capable as before his illness. Prior to his illness, Harry was an avid golfer, loved to cook, loved to drive, and volunteered in community activities. After his diagnosis and treatment, Shirley decided that Harry was no longer capable of driving and cooking. She also wanted him to cut back on his golf and community activities. Staying home and resting were the activities she felt were in his best interest. Shirley's good intentions caused Harry to feel more depressed, until he rebelled. He took control by asserting himself.

Shirley and Harry are an example of a very common problem. Often patients are discouraged from leading an active lifestyle and maintaining a normal routine. The misconception is that if you have cancer, you are incapacitated or need to conserve your energy in order to prevent speeding up the process of your disease. Most patients benefit from maintaining as normal a life as they possibly can. Tom's case illustrates this point.

Tom had an advanced case of stomach cancer. He experienced pain, depression, anxiety, insomnia, and loss of appetite. Nevertheless, his oncologist recommended that he go back to work and begin exercising again. Tom wanted to return to work and reported that whenever he was active, he experienced less pain and depression. However, Tom's wife expressed her fear that his condition would worsen if he did not remain in bed. Both Dr. Bill Golden and Tom's oncologist told his wife that activity would not harm him. Bill also explained that when cancer patients are active they enjoy a better quality of life and may even live longer than patients who are passive. Tom's wife accepted this explanation and cooperated with his activity program. Activities such as mild exercise, swimming, doing chores, and visiting friends were encouraged. These activities significantly reduced Tom's depression and some of his pain. He eventually returned to work and received a promotion. Although he died two and a half years later, he enjoyed an active, productive lifestyle prior to his last hospitalization.

These examples of good intentions encouraging helplessness seem to occur without warning. Most of our patients have said that when they are treated this way they feel "foolish" and "useless," and have remarked to us: "This is so unfair—my doctor said I have no limitations." Mel remarked that when he was trying to help pack his car for a vacation he felt like he was being ignored—as if he wasn't there. Everybody was packing the car and prevented him from contributing. Mel said, "I felt like I didn't exist."

Mel needed to learn to be assertive. However, because his family's behavior occurred so unexpectedly, he was caught off guard and didn't know how to respond. In discussing this situation with his psychologist, Dr. David Robbins, he learned that all he needed to do was not participate as a helpless person, but instead to become assertive. David shared his own similar experiences and said, "My family would do anything to help me, but initially they made the same mistakes. Just about everyone falls into the same trap. I told them that I'm not helpless. On the contrary, I'm quite capable, and I want the opportunity to do as much as I can because it will make me feel better. You can do the same thing. Just be assertive with them, not hostile. Talk to them in a calm but assertive manner. By being assertive and calm, you will be more likely to get them to treat you the way you want."

As you can see, these examples demonstrate how assertiveness can remedy the problem of possibly harmful good intentions. Keep in mind the principles of assertiveness discussed in chapter 7: Don't attack your friends and family members. Don't blame them. Don't say, "You make me feel helpless." Take responsibility for your feelings. Express how you feel using "I" statements. For example, "I feel helpless when you do things for me that I could do myself." Make suggestions and tell them what you would like them to do instead. For example, "I would like to help pack the car." You could acknowledge their good intentions. For example, "I appreciate your wanting to do this for me, but I'm quite capable of participating." Remember, the goal is to be assertive and not hostile. So be calm, be brief, and avoid hostilities.

Responding to Others' Inappropriate Remarks

Worse than being treated like a helpless person is being treated as if you were already dead. This problem is not that common be-

cause family members tend to hide their feelings about your illness as part of the web of silence. Nevertheless, several of our
patients have reported being treated by family, friends, and physicians as if they were hopeless cases or already dead. Nothing
could be more demoralizing than being treated as if you were
about to die.

Every time Mary's husband looked at her, his eyes teared up
and he would repeatedly ask, "How will I go on without you?
How will I manage the house? Who will help me with the kids?"
Finally, as a result of counseling, Mary learned to be assertive. She
was able to acknowledge her husband's feelings, yet tell him how
she was affected. "I know you're very worried about how you're
going to manage, but it's really upsetting to hear you talk about
me as if I were already dead."

Phil was in the hospital getting chemotherapy. When his divorced parents came to visit him, he was lying in bed recovering
from his treatment. His parents took up positions on opposite sides
of his bed and proceeded to argue about what they would do with
Phil's possessions when he died. Phil reported to Dr. David Robbins that he felt like he wasn't there, like he was being written off
by his parents, and that his feelings didn't count. Phil was assertive
enough to be able to express his feelings to his parents. When his
parents were arguing about the division of his estate in front of
him, Phil was able to say, "Stop this! Get out of my room—I'm
going to survive." Eight years later, Phil was still alive.

Physicians can sometimes inadvertently convey the message
that your case is hopeless. Phil was told by his physician that he
had only six months to live. Mat, who had esophageal cancer, was
also told by his surgeon, "Don't sign any long-term mortgages."
Neither of these physicians intended to harm or demoralize these
patients. Unfortunately, physicians and other health care workers
are in a precarious position. They are often not certain as to what
the patient needs to hear versus what the patient wants to hear.
In the past, the common practice was to tell cancer patients as
little as possible about their diagnosis and prognosis. Then, the
pendulum swung in the opposite direction, so that physicians felt
required to tell patients everything, whether the patient wanted to
hear this information or not. We now know that there are at least
three groups of patients: Some patients want to know as much as
possible about their diagnosis, prognosis, and medical procedures.
Other patients prefer (and do better) knowing nothing—or as little

as possible. A third group of patients seek information about their diagnosis and medical procedures, but are not interested in the physician's prognostic predictions.

To which group do you belong? What kind of information do you want to get from your physician, and what information do you not want to hear? A word of caution: Keep in mind that the problem with receiving a prognosis is that it can become self-fulfilling. A self-fulfilling prophecy is one that you "live up to" or "die down to." You don't have to accept any prophecies. Remember: Accept the diagnosis, but defy the prognosis.

You have several alternatives if you should find yourself in a situation where your physician is giving you information and predictions that you don't want to hear. Being assertive is one alternative. You can say to your physician, "I really would prefer that you don't tell me all that you know about my illness." For some of you this might be an extremely difficult thing to say because we tend to deify our physicians. Keep in mind that you are a consumer. A patient is a consumer of medical services, and a physician is the provider of these services. Don't feel intimidated. Your physician is a human being, just like you. Don't be afraid of being abandoned or receiving inadequate services. We have never heard of a physician abandoning a patient for being assertive. At the very worst, your physician could get defensive and not be receptive. This makes him or her just like any other human being.

Despite our advice that you speak up, you may still be apprehensive. You have other options. You don't have to confront your physician. You might be able to tell your spouse or friend to tell the physician that you really don't want as much information as the physician is telling you. Another option is to treat the prognosis as an opinion. It's not written in stone. Keep in mind the people we have described, or perhaps people you know, who have lived well past their physicians' predictions.

Physicians are not the only people who can make remarks that are well intentioned but are hurtful. They can come from anyone at anytime. Friends and relatives can make hurtful remarks. Shortly after surgery, David, the third author, met an acquaintance who noticed the scar on his head and came up with the following thoughtless remark: "I see you've had surgery. Stan's brother had the same surgery and he died." David was left feeling empty. Despite being a psychologist and being able to deal with many other types of thoughtless remarks, this one really got to him. This was only the first of a long series of thoughtless remarks made by many other people in David's life. David decided that it wasn't important enough to be assertive with everyone who made these remarks. He decided to pick and choose with whom to be assertive. He felt that being assertive with everyone would have taken more time and energy than it was worth. Instead, he decided to spend his time with people who were not so callous. He also found that he spent more time alone, enjoying his own company. In addition, he even learned to see the humor in people who have the knack for saying exactly the wrong thing at the wrong time.

Like David, you may find yourself bombarded with people who make thoughtless remarks. Again, you have choices as to how you may want to respond. Being assertive is certainly one option. You can say to them, "You probably don't realize it, but what you just said was not appreciated." Don't be surprised if you get a lot of strange reactions to your being assertive. We are talking about people who are prone to being inappropriate. So don't expect an appropriate reaction to your assertiveness. There are always at least two reasons for being assertive. One, you may get an appropriate response such as an apology. The other reason for being assertive is for your own mental health. Being assertive can be cathartic and can promote feelings of self-respect. You can also choose, as David did, not to say anything to these people. You may feel as he did, that your time and energy should not be wasted with people who don't think. The way to minimize the hurt is to mentally prepare yourself for these comments. Tell yourself, "I know people will make these comments, but I can deal with them. I don't have to dwell on negative remarks. There are more important issues to focus on."

Sometimes a caring, thoughtful person can make a thoughtless remark. That person might even be very close to you, like a spouse, family member, or friend. Telling them how you feel is very important because if you don't, they can continue to make such remarks and you can develop resentment. Expressing your feelings can strengthen the relationship. Be assertive rather than hostile, because you don't want to alienate your support system if it can be avoided. Express your hurt or other feelings using the assertiveness guidelines described earlier.

You are more likely to be assertive as opposed to hostile if you reduce your anger. It's understandable that you would feel anger toward a person who makes an unkind remark. It's natural that you would feel more hurt and betrayed when that person is

> *Expecting your loved ones or friends to be perfect and always say the right thing is not realistic.*

a loved one. Although anger is a natural response to these situations, expressing it in a nonconstructive manner will be neither beneficial nor helpful. Therefore, reducing anger to a manageable level allows you the best opportunity to express it constructively. Expecting your loved ones or friends to be perfect and to always say the right thing is not realistic. Expect them to be human. From time to time, even people who love you or care about you will say and do the wrong thing. Expect it—but you don't have to accept it. Without condemning them, tell people how you feel.

It is important to be assertive not only to let people know when they have done something wrong, but also to encourage them to do things right. Use the exercise below to improve your assertiveness in asking for and getting the support you need from the people around you.

Your Support Plan

Use the form below to list people you need to ask for help and support, and what you should say to them.

Potential Supporter	What to Say

When you finish listing potential supporters, pick the easiest one to try first. Practice asking for support out loud, role-playing the scene with a friend. Or you can imagine the conversation first in your mind's eye. Pick an appropriate time, and ask the most approachable person on your list for the help you need. Success with the easiest person on your list will give you practice and confidence to approach the more challenging people.

When Lynne made her support plan, she focused on three people: her husband, George; her friend, Jan; and her boss:

Potential Supporter	What to Say
George	*I don't have my old energy any more. I need you to come home on time each night and help with the housework. And I'd really like you to spend time with me on Saturday mornings instead of seeing clients.*
Jan	*Could you help me find a home for Cocoa? I can't walk a dog every day, and George doesn't have time for her either.*
Boss	*I know the employee manual says an employee on leave can't take vacation time as pay, but I really need the money and I would like you to make an exception.*

Lynne talked to her boss first, then to Jan. Those conversations went okay, so she approached her husband next. By being calm and persistent, she was able to break through his denial, show him that her cancer required both of them to make adjustments, and get the support she needed to conserve her energy and maintain her quality of life.

Sex

Another aspect of reaching out is the resurrection of sexual intimacy. This involves breaking down sexual inhibitions that frequently develop after a diagnosis of cancer. Loss of sexual drive, changes in self-esteem, and negative feelings about one's body are frequently occurring problems. They can result from the illness or its treatments, such as radiation, chemotherapy, or surgery.

The reason you may be experiencing a decrease of sexual drive is due either to physical or biochemical changes that can occur from treatment, or to emotional reactions. Anxiety and depression can decrease your interest in sex. Embarrassment or anxiety about changes in your physical appearance can likewise inhibit sexuality. We will address the emotional side of the problem. We recommend that you consult your physician about possible sexual side effects that can occur from your medical treatments. Discuss with your physician the possible interventions that may be available. For example, chemotherapy for Hodgkin's disease may cause a loss of sexual desire. However, hormone replacement therapy can result in a return to normal sexual function. Your physician may also be able to reassure you that the side effects you are experiencing are temporary.

For other sexual difficulties, such as painful intercourse following surgery, sexual counseling may be helpful. Sometimes simple interventions can provide relief. For example, a shortened vagina resulting from surgery can produce painful intercourse. Avoiding deep penile thrusting can alleviate the problem. Experimenting with more comfortable positions can be a solution, such as elevating the woman's buttocks with a pillow during intercourse. Another example of a simple intervention involves the use of lubricants for patients who have difficulties with natural vaginal lubrication. Of course, open and honest communication is of paramount importance. You and your partner need to be able to talk openly about your physical problems as well as your feelings in order to overcome these difficulties.

Loss of self-esteem frequently occurs as a result of changes in one's body image. After surgery that causes distinct changes in anatomy, you may experience profound emotional distress. A large part of the emotional distress concerns fear about sexual rejection. You may feel that your partner, who was attracted to you prior to your surgery, will now find you undesirable. Because of your altered body image, you may believe that you are ugly. You may feel too ashamed or scared to approach your partner to discuss his or her feelings. In chapter 7, we presented methods for achieving self-acceptance despite rejection and disapproval. Let's apply those techniques to your fear of sexual rejection and loss of self-esteem.

Although your body has undergone real changes that cannot be denied, you can still see yourself as a desirable, attractive, sexual being. Instead of focusing on your physical changes, focus on what is still beautiful and desirable about you. Don't generalize. You are not just a breast, a vagina, a penis, or a pretty face. You are more than the sum of your parts. Your partner did not fall in love with you just for your breast, your vagina, your penis, or your pretty face. Both you and your partner can highlight and emphasize your desirable features. Both of you have the choice of looking at the glass as half empty or half full. Obviously, you will find yourself more desirable, your partner will find you more desirable, and you will be more sexual if the positives are emphasized.

Don't allow yourself to believe that beauty is only what the media tells you. For example, breasts have been idealized in this culture. Your sexuality is not negated because of a mastectomy. For example, Rebecca, a single woman, thought she was no longer attractive after her mastectomy. Although she had several reconstructive surgeries, none of them were able to make her breast look natural. She was afraid to date men because she felt that if the relationship became sexual, she would be rejected. She was convinced that her breast was ugly and deformed.

Rebecca came to counseling with Dr. Wayne Gersh because she was lonely and depressed. She was in conflict. Her goal was to have a relationship, but she was terrified of rejection. She was convinced that no man would want her. Wayne explained that, in his experience, most men still find their wives attractive despite a mastectomy, whether or not reconstructive surgery has occurred.

Rebecca objected: "But those women were already married. It's a lot different for me. I don't have a boyfriend."

Wayne agreed, "It is a lot harder for a single woman. I do know of at least one case involving a single, unattached woman. She was also afraid of rejection, but I helped her to take risks and eventually she met somebody. What I recommended to her, and what I recommend to you, is that you allow the guy to get to know you. Once someone knows you as a person, they are less likely to reject you when they find out about your surgery."

"Well, that's only one case," said Rebecca.

Wayne then asked Rebecca, "Have you heard of Betty Rollin?"

"No. I don't know who she is," Rebecca responded.

Wayne described Betty Rollin's story and told Rebecca about her book, First You Cry (1993). Betty Rollin had a double mastectomy. At first she felt "de-womanized." She had reconstructive surgery that involved saline implants in both breasts. Eventually, she felt good about herself again, feeling proud of herself as a survivor. She divorced her first husband after her first breast surgery, met a "great" man, and married him. Wayne suggested, "I think you would find this book very helpful. I recommend that you read it so that you can get a woman's perspective."

Rebecca returned the following week having read the book. She had become receptive to working on her problem. Wayne encouraged Rebecca to start taking risks and begin socializing. In working on her anxiety about rejection, he focused on getting Rebecca to accept herself despite rejection. She learned how to focus on her positive attributes as a way of reducing low self-esteem. For example, Rebecca listed positives such as her pretty eyes, shapely legs, and wonderful smile. She noted her sophistication, the success she'd had in her career, and her warm, caring, and sensitive personality. And finally, that she was very proud to be a survivor.

She began dating and eventually met a man she liked who also liked her. After several dates, when it looked like the relationship could progress, Rebecca became terrified. She came to her next counseling session not knowing what to do. She felt like ending the relationship: "I'd rather just end it and avoid the pain of rejection."

Wayne asked, "How do you know he will reject you?"

"I'm just not willing to take the chance," said Rebecca.

Wayne said, "Then we can be sure that you will never have a relationship. What happened to your goal?"

"Well, then what should I do?" she asked.

Wayne advised, "First of all, you are assuming rejection. Everything you have told me about this man makes me think that he will accept you. But even if he rejects you, that does not make you less worthwhile or less of a woman. As long as you continue to take risks, you will eventually have the relationship that you want. So, go out with him and let the relationship progress."

Rebecca took Wayne's advice and continued to date this man. He was completely accepting about her surgery and encouraged her to feel good about herself. Eventually, she felt good about his seeing and touching her breasts, and they were able to develop a mutually satisfying sexual relationship. Ironically, Rebecca reported that this was her best relationship ever, and that she was having the best sex she had ever had.

Men can also have sexual difficulties as a result of cancer. For example, men can have altered sexual functioning from medical procedures such as a prostectomy. Nevertheless, sexuality does not have to end. Sex is not just intercourse. Society places too much of an emphasis on obtaining sexual gratification through intercourse. Even if there is loss of sexual functioning for medical reasons, you still can give and get pleasure manually and orally.

Eric sought counseling from Dr. Bill Golden because he felt inadequate after his prostectomy. He could no longer obtain an erection and discontinued all sexual contact with his wife. He said,

"I'm not a man anymore. I can't get an erection. I can't please my wife, so what's the use?"

Bill asked, "Have you considered getting a penile implant operation? Do you know what that is?"

Eric said, "That's too artificial, and besides, I've had enough surgery for now."

"Have you and your wife tried doing other things, like oral sex?" asked Bill.

"But what's the point if I can't get it up? Sex is too upsetting. It's just a reminder that I'm not the same. It's just not the same anymore."

Bill asked, "What is your wife's reaction to all of this?" Eric reported that his wife was very frustrated because he was unwilling to go for a penile implant operation, nor would he hug, kiss, or touch her. She wasn't being demanding and said whatever Eric decided about the penile implant operation was fine with her. She just wanted to be hugged and held, and she wanted him to feel good about himself.

Bill acknowledged Eric's frustration. "This is a real hard thing for most men to accept. The natural tendency is to shy away from all sex. But you're still capable of giving and receiving pleasure. It's important to continue to have sexual intimacy in whatever form you and your wife are able to experience. I'm sure we'll be able to figure out something that would be acceptable for you and your wife. But before we do that, we need to work on your feelings about yourself. You're putting yourself down and no longer thinking of yourself as a man. You are still a man. Don't equate your manhood with your ability to get an erection. You can still please your wife manually and orally. If you accept yourself and accept what you can do, you'll feel better about yourself."

Eric realized that he was being too tough on himself and not allowing himself any options. He agreed to work on changing his attitudes about himself and his sexuality. Over several weeks of counseling, Eric became more self-accepting. At that point, he brought his wife to counseling. They agreed to postpone the decision about Eric getting a penile implant. A penile implant operation would allow him to get an erection, but he was willing to wait. They were willing to come to counseling to learn other ways to interact sexually. As their counseling progressed, both Eric and his wife reported a renewed interest and greater satisfaction in sex.

Reaching out involves taking risks, being assertive, and working on self-acceptance. You may find it difficult taking these risks and being assertive. It is hard because it involves learning new behavior and confronting fear. Don't let this discourage you. Risk taking gets easier with time and practice. Assertiveness and communication are skills that develop over time. Most people find it hard to talk about intimate feelings, especially those involving sexuality. If you persist and confront your fears, you will find that reaching out was well worth the risk. Your life will become much richer.

Support Groups

As mentioned previously in this book, Dr. David Spiegel's research has shown that supportive group therapy improved the quality of life of patients and may even have helped them to survive their cancer for a greater length of time. He speculates that although there were a number of therapeutic interventions used in those groups, what may have been most important was the emotional support that the group members received from one another.

Take some time to consider joining a self-help group. Use the list of resources at the end of this book to locate organizations that provide groups you can join. Sometimes there are groups run by the hospital where you've been treated. These may be support groups, or art therapy, relaxation therapy, or general information groups.

In addition, there are groups that will help you in learning how to cope with life after chemotherapy or other forms of treatment. Almost every hospital has a support group for you and your family. Typically, there are support groups for every form of cancer that the hospital treats. Sometimes these group meetings are posted in the outpatient department as well as the inpatient units. Calling the social services department of the hospital should give you the information you would need to contact the group you are interested in attending.

Support groups are also offered by the American Cancer Society (ACS). These groups can help you with psychological issues, such as coping with anxiety and depression, as well as teaching you how to manage your illness. This may include learning how to wear a wig or a prosthetic device. Some of these groups run by the American Cancer Society have what is called "A Day of Beauty." Cosmetic and wig companies offer their expertise and samples of their products.

> *She came back to her counseling session saying*
> *that she was amazed at how good she looked*
> *and felt from the cosmetic consultation.*

One of our patients, Wendy, was exuberant after her day of beauty. She told us to tell all of our patients about her experience. Initially, she was feeling depressed because she thought she was unattractive as a result of her chemotherapy treatment. She was losing her hair, and her complexion was pale from the treatments. At first, she was reluctant about going to her beauty day. She was very skeptical about how a wig and cosmetics could possibly make her look attractive again. She came back to her counseling session saying that she was amazed at how good she looked and felt from the cosmetic consultation. The cosmetic company gave her what seemed to be hundreds of dollars worth of makeup. A cosmetologist from the company was present to give the cancer support group members advice about how to look their best, despite the effects of chemotherapy. "I thought I knew how to apply makeup, but after the chemotherapy, no matter what I tried I still looked ugly. I felt so frustrated and depressed. After a while, I stopped trying. Look at me now. I feel like myself again!"

Wendy also was pleasantly surprised about the wigs. At first she was reluctant to even try one because she thought it would make her look fake. However, the wig company that came to her support group provided her with a blonde, a brunette, and an auburn wig. She had fun trying them on and began to enjoy the variety. Some days she wears the brunette one, and other days she gets a kick out of being a blonde.

Similar to the hospital groups, the groups from the ACS are differentiated by the type of cancer you have. Even if your local ACS chapter does not offer a support group for your type of cancer, they will be able to direct you to groups or individuals who do. For example, professionals such as the authors of this book can be an excellent resource for these types of groups.

Other supportive services that the ACS can offer include financial help for treatment, home care workers, or transportation to and from treatments. For example, Dr. David Robbins needed transportation to his radiation treatments. He lives in a community that is many miles from the hospital where these treatments were to take place. He first reached out to family and friends, but quickly realized that this was not an adequate solution since the people in his life were not available at the time he needed to go for treatment. His wife suggested that he call the ACS, and he told them of his predicament. They provided David with a driver who was able to get him to treatment for a fee of twenty dollars. The interesting sidelight to this story was that when David went to pay for this service, his driver would not take any money. He informed David that he too was a cancer patient and that when he needed a driver, he was not charged. Therefore, he was not going to take any money from David.

There are different types and functions of support groups. Some of these groups can provide patients with an opportunity to express their thoughts and feelings about their illness and their future. A lot of networking also takes place. Patients exchange information about other treatments, specialists, support groups, and other services. Some support groups are more informational. For example, a group given at Community Hospital in Dobbs Ferry, New York, brought together a number of cancer specialists. The specialists provided information about treatments, their benefits, and their side effects. Dr. Wayne Gersh participated in the program. He taught the members of the support group techniques for coping with cancer. One of the most important techniques taught was relaxation and deep breathing. The members reported feeling significantly more relaxed and felt that this was a technique they would continue to use.

> *Support groups provide you with a forum to express feelings and thoughts that you might not feel comfortable expressing to friends and family members.*

There are a number of benefits to support groups. As we mentioned earlier, research conducted by Dr. David Spiegel and his associates has shown that support groups led to improved quality of life and in some cases longer periods of survival. Many of our patients report that they find comfort in support groups. They feel that by sharing feelings with other people who are going through the same experiences, they feel less isolated and less alone. Support groups provide you with a forum to express feelings and thoughts that you might not feel comfortable expressing to friends and family members. Many of our patients say that when they express their fears and doubts to friends and family members they are often given well-intentioned advice. There is a time and place for advice and techniques. However, advice and techniques may not be what you want at that moment. Sometimes you may just want to get things off your chest and be heard. Friends and family members don't realize that being supportive sometimes means just listening. In support groups, feelings are validated. Validation of feelings involves listening without critical evaluation. There is instead empathy and compassion.

Support groups aren't for everyone. Some people find them depressing. A lot of intense emotion is expressed in a support group, and whereas some people find expressing emotions to be cathartic, other people experience it as negative. Sometimes it's not easy or comfortable to be confronted with your fears and doubts. Some people prefer not to express those feelings and instead prefer to focus on positive thinking and problem solving exclusively. You have the right to decide what is the appropriate supportive environment for you.

Another reason why support groups might not be for you is that some people don't feel comfortable sharing in a group setting. Some patients are just not "group therapy people" and are more comfortable with individual counseling. Again, it's important to choose the right venue for you.

A potential problem with support groups is that the group may become dominated by one or two of its members. This problem is most likely to occur in groups without a leader or in groups where the leader is too passive. More active leaders will intervene when a member has a tendency to dominate or be abusive to other members. If you find that you are uncomfortable in a particular support group, then trust your feelings and find a different group. Not all groups are the same. Pick the one that's right for you.

Online Support

Perhaps you've tried to find a support group and found that there were none available in your area. If you have a computer, you are only a keystroke away from a supportive network. All you need is to obtain software that will connect you to the Internet. Once connected, you can begin searching for material or information about your illness. You can also connect with other people who have the same or similar cancer as yours.

> *If you have a computer, you are only a keystroke away from a supportive network.*

Michael, one of Dr. Wayne Gersh's patients, was diagnosed as having a rare lymphoma. He was one of those individuals who did not like groups. Yet he had the need to communicate with others about his illness. He also was confused about the number of treatment choices that were available to him. His doctors told him that the ultimate decision as to which treatment to pursue was his. They did not have any patient education information to give him that would assist him in making his decision. Wayne recommended that Michael use his computer to access the Internet to see if he could discover information about his illness. Michael came back to his counseling session with many pages of information about research on all the treatments for his illness. In addition, he used chat rooms and bulletin boards to communicate with people who were going through the various treatments. He heard about their personal experiences, including their side effects, frustrations, and successes. He and Wayne were then able to discuss the advantages and disadvantages of each treatment, enabling Michael to arrive at a decision.

Michael also used the Internet to cope with some of the frustrations he experienced while undergoing his treatment. For example, he was quite discouraged when his physician told him that he needed to continue the treatment for a longer period of time than was originally projected. He started to lose faith in his physician and his treatment. He was confused about what to do. Should he try one of the other treatments? As a result of networking on the Internet, he found other people who needed a more prolonged period of treatment and who, in the end, did respond favorably. This gave him the faith to continue.

Sometimes meaningful relationships can be developed through the Internet. Patients who have never met each other can and do form strong emotional bonds. Many of our patients have reported that they communicate on a regular basis with friends they have met on the Internet. Using e-mail is an effective way to keep in touch with other people who share similar interests and concerns.

Jane began using the Internet to find other people who were diagnosed with a brain tumor known as glioblastoma. She was

> *Sometimes meaningful relationships*
> *can be developed through the Internet.*
> *Patients who have never met each other*
> *can and do form strong emotional bonds.*

very fortunate in locating a site designated for individuals with brain tumors. It was further differentiated into a site for glioblastomas. At that point, Jane left her e-mail address. Another patient using the same bulletin board responded to her request for interaction, and a correspondence was begun. Jane started by sharing treatment information. Eventually, the correspondence became more intimate. Jane and her correspondent discussed their families, their musical interests, other hobbies, and their fears. A strong emotional bond was developed, even though they never met.

There are some other things that you can do for additional help. There are limits to self-help procedures and support groups. Some problems are serious and require professional help. There are psychologists, such as ourselves, who specialize in the treatment of cancer patients. We feel that professionals who counsel cancer patients should have a cognitive-behavioral background. Cognitive-behavior therapy is the most effective treatment for the problems associated with cancer. There is extensive research that shows that cognitive-behavior therapy is effective in the treatment of depression, anxiety, stress, pain, and the trauma associated with medical procedures.

When we began writing this book, we felt that our goal was to reach a larger audience than we were capable of reaching in our private practice. We wanted to share the tools that were benefiting so many of our patients. We have seen people who would have given up if they did not have the benefit of the methods we have detailed here. Some of these individuals actually encouraged us to write this book so that others could benefit from the methods that had improved their lives.

You can learn to use these techniques on your own. We know it's possible because our patients have shared our techniques and tapes with other cancer patients—with great success. These other patients were helped even though they did not see us. You can do it too! We wish you good luck and hope that you have found our book both helpful and inspirational.

Organizations Providing Assistance for Cancer Patients

- **American Cancer Society**
  1-800-ACS-2345
  Tower Place
  3340 Peachtree Road NE
  Atlanta, GA 30026

This well-known organization has chapters in most communities. They provide assistance in obtaining information about cancer and will assist in helping patients utilize community resources and obtain aids such as wigs and prosthetic devices. The American Cancer Society will also arrange transportation, lend and rent equipment, and provide small stipends if money is needed. Patient services include support groups for many different forms of cancer.

- **Cancer Care, Inc.**
  212-221-3300
  1180 Avenue of the Americas
  New York, NY 10036

This is an organization that provides free counseling for cancer patients and their families. These services are available in New York, New Jersey, and Connecticut. Patients in other areas of the country can call Cancer Care to obtain a list of organizations that will provide similar services in their area. They will also provide written information upon request.

- Cancer Information Service
1-800-4-CANCER

The Cancer Information Service provides information about cancer to patients and their families. Education is provided about the latest treatments for cancer, risk factors, and early detection. They offer information on community resources and can provide written information about the illness upon request.

- Corporate Angel Network
914-328-1313
Westchester County Airport
White Plains, NY 10604

Corporate Angel Network provides patients with air transportation on corporate jets to National Cancer Institute–approved treatment facilities.

- The National Coalition of Cancer Survivorship
301-650-8868
1010 Wayne Avenue, Fifth Floor
Silver Spring, MD 20910

This is a network of individuals and organizations who serve as advocates for cancer patients and their families. They help patients and their families obtain services. They also provide peer support and information.

References

Benson, H. 1996. *Timeless Healing*. New York: Fireside-Simon & Schuster.

Burns, D. 1984. *Feeling Good: The New Mood Therapy*. New York: William Morrow.

Cousins, N. 1989. *Head First: The Biology of Hope*. New York: E. P. Dutton.

Ellis, A., and R. Harper. 1975. *A New Guide to Rational Living*. North Hollywood, CA: Wilshire.

Fawzy, F., N. Fawzy, R. Hynn, D. Elashott, J. Guthrie, J. Fahey, and D. Morton. 1993. Malignant melanoma: Effects of an early structured psychiatric intervention, coping and affective state on recurrence and survival 6 years later. *Archives of General Psychiatry* 50:681–689.

Fensterheim, H., and J. Baer. 1975. *Don't Say Yes When You Want to Say No*. New York: David McKay.

Golden, W., E. Dowd, and F. Friedberg. 1987. *Hypnotherapy: A Modern Approach*. New York: Pergamon Press.

Golden, W., W. Gersh, and D. Robbins. 1992. *Psychological Treatment of Cancer Patients: A Cognitive-Behavioral Approach*. Needham Heights, MA: Allyn and Bacon.

Gruber, B., N. Hall, S. Hersh, and P. Dubois. 1988. Immune system and psychologic changes in metastatic cancer patients while using ritualized relaxation and guided imagery: A pilot study. *Scandinavian Journal of Behavior Therapy* 17:25–46.

International Association for the Study of Pain. 1979. Subcommittee on Taxonomy Pain Terms: A List with Definitions and Notes on Usage. *Pain.* 6:249–252.

Kubler-Ross, E. 1969. *On Death and Dying.* New York: Macmillan.

Le Shan, L. 1977. *You Can Fight for Your Life.* New York: Evans.

Rollin, B. 1993. *First You Cry.* New York: Harper Collins.

Spiegel, D. 1993. *Living Beyond Limits: New Hope for Facing Life-Threatening Illness.* New York: Times Books.

Wolpe, J. 1958. *Psychotherapy by Reciprocal Inhibition.* Stanford, CA: Stanford University.

The above list of readings and references is only a partial list of the resources that we used in writing this book. For a more complete list of references, refer to our textbook, *Psychological Treatment of Cancer Patients: A Cognitive-Behavioral Approach.*

Index

Many people find that the best way to learn relaxation and self-hypnosis is by listening to cassette tapes of these procedures. Throughout the book we have described how you can make your own tapes using the various relaxation and self-hypnosis transcripts. If you would prefer a professionally made tape, contact us at:

Dr. Wayne Gersh, Dr. William Golden, and Dr. David Robbins
Westchester Center for Behavior Therapy
77 Tarrytown Road
White Plains, NY 10607

More New Harbinger Titles

THE CHEMOTHERAPY SURVIVAL GUIDE
Explains how chemotherapy works and tells you exactly what you can do to prevent or minimize side-effects. *Item CHEM Paperback $11.95*

THE DAILY RELAXER
Presents the most effective and popular techniques for learning how to relax—simple, tension-relieving exercises that you can learn in five minutes and practice with positive results right away.
Item DALY Paperback, $12.95

THE CHRONIC PAIN CONTROL WORKBOOK
A team of specialists in all areas of pain management detail the treatment strategies for managing and recovering from chronic pain.
Item PN2 Paperback $17.95

THE DEPRESSION WORKBOOK
Interactive exercises teach essential coping skills. Based on the responses of 120 survey participants who share their strategies for living with extreme mood swings. *Item DEP Paperback $17.95*

THE THREE MINUTE MEDITATOR
The expanded third edition offers a down-to-earth introduction to the basics of using meditation to unwind your mind, cope with the stresses of daily life, and treat yourself to the powerful benefits of self-acceptance and inner peace. *Item MED3 Paperback, $12.95*

FIBROMYALGIA & CHRONIC MYOFASCIAL PAIN SYNDROME
This survival manual is the first comprehensive patient guide for managing these conditions. Readers learn how to identify trigger points, cope with chronic pain and sleep problems, and deal with the numbing effects of "fibrofog." *Item FMS Paperback, $19.95*

Call **toll-free 1-800-748-6273** to order. Have your Visa or Mastercard number ready. Or send a check for the titles you want to New Harbinger Publications, 5674 Shattuck Avenue, Oakland, CA 94609. Include $3.80 for the first book and 75¢ for each additional book to cover shipping and handling. (California residents please include appropriate sales tax.) Allow four to six weeks for delivery.

Prices subject to change without notice.

Other New Harbinger Self-Help Titles

Ten Things Every Parent Needs to Know, $12.95
The Power of Two, $12.95
It's Not OK Anymore, $13.95
The Daily Relaxer, $12.95
The Body Image Workbook, $17.95
Living with ADD, $17.95
Taking the Anxiety Out of Taking Tests, $12.95
The Taking Charge of Menopause Workbook, $17.95
Living with Angina, $12.95
PMS: Women Tell Women How to Control Premenstrual Syndrome, $13.95
Five Weeks to Healing Stress: The Wellness Option, $17.95
Choosing to Live: How to Defeat Suicide Through Cognitive Therapy, $12.95
Why Children Misbehave and What to Do About It, $14.95
Illuminating the Heart, $13.95
When Anger Hurts Your Kids, $12.95
The Addiction Workbook, $17.95
The Mother's Survival Guide to Recovery, $12.95
The Chronic Pain Control Workbook, Second Edition, $17.95
Fibromyalgia & Chronic Myofascial Pain Syndrome, $19.95
Diagnosis and Treatment of Sociopaths, $44.95
Flying Without Fear, $12.95
Kid Cooperation: How to Stop Yelling, Nagging & Pleading and Get Kids to Cooperate, $12.95
The Stop Smoking Workbook: Your Guide to Healthy Quitting, $17.95
Conquering Carpal Tunnel Syndrome and Other Repetitive Strain Injuries, $17.95
The Tao of Conversation, $12.95
Wellness at Work: Building Resilience for Job Stress, $17.95
What Your Doctor Can't Tell You About Cosmetic Surgery, $13.95
An End to Panic: Breakthrough Techniques for Overcoming Panic Disorder, $17.95
On the Clients Path: A Manual for the Practice of Solution-Focused Therapy, $39.95
Living Without Procrastination: How to Stop Postponing Your Life, $12.95
Goodbye Mother, Hello Woman: Reweaving the Daughter Mother Relationship, $14.95
Letting Go of Anger: The 10 Most Common Anger Styles and What to Do About Them, $12.95
Messages: The Communication Skills Workbook, Second Edition, $13.95
Coping With Chronic Fatigue Syndrome: Nine Things You Can Do, $12.95
The Anxiety & Phobia Workbook, Second Edition, $17.95
Thueson's Guide to Over-the-Counter Drugs, $13.95
Natural Women's Health: A Guide to Healthy Living for Women of Any Age, $13.95
I'd Rather Be Married: Finding Your Future Spouse, $13.95
The Relaxation & Stress Reduction Workbook, Fourth Edition, $17.95
Living Without Depression & Manic Depression: A Workbook for Maintaining Mood Stability, $17.95
Belonging: A Guide to Overcoming Loneliness, $13.95
Coping With Schizophrenia: A Guide For Families, $13.95
Visualization for Change, Second Edition, $13.95
Postpartum Survival Guide, $13.95
Angry All the Time: An Emergency Guide to Anger Control, $12.95
Couple Skills: Making Your Relationship Work, $13.95
Handbook of Clinical Psychopharmacology for Therapists, $39.95
Weight Loss Through Persistence, $13.95
Post-Traumatic Stress Disorder: A Complete Treatment Guide, $39.95
Stepfamily Realities: How to Overcome Difficulties and Have a Happy Family, $13.95
The Chemotherapy Survival Guide, $11.95
Your Family/Your Self: How to Analyze Your Family System, $12.95
The Deadly Diet, Second Edition: Recovering from Anorexia & Bulimia, $13.95
Last Touch: Preparing for a Parent's Death, $11.95
Self-Esteem, Second Edition, $13.95
I Can't Get Over It, A Handbook for Trauma Survivors, Second Edition, $15.95
Concerned Intervention, When Your Loved One Won't Quit Alcohol or Drugs, $12.95
Dying of Embarrassment: Help for Social Anxiety and Social Phobia, $12.95
The Depression Workbook: Living With Depression and Manic Depression, $17.95
Prisoners of Belief: Exposing & Changing Beliefs that Control Your Life, $12.95
Men & Grief: A Guide for Men Surviving the Death of a Loved One, $13.95
When the Bough Breaks: A Helping Guide for Parents of Sexually Abused Children, $11.95
When Once Is Not Enough: Help for Obsessive Compulsives, $13.95
The Three Minute Meditator, Third Edition, $12.95
Beyond Grief: A Guide for Recovering from the Death of a Loved One, $13.95
Leader's Guide to the Relaxation & Stress Reduction Workbook, Fourth Edition, $19.95
The Divorce Book, $13.95
Hypnosis for Change: A Manual of Proven Techniques, Third Edition, $13.95
When Anger Hurts, $13.95
Lifetime Weight Control, $12.95

Call **toll free, 1-800-748-6273,** to order. Have your Visa or Mastercard number ready. Or send a check for the titles you want to New Harbinger Publications, Inc., 5674 Shattuck Ave., Oakland, CA 94609. Include $3.80 for the first book and 75¢ for each additional book, to cover shipping and handling. (California residents please include appropriate sales tax.) Allow four to six weeks for delivery.

Prices subject to change without notice.